HEALTH SERVICES PERFORMANCE

HEALTH SERVICES PERFORMANCE

Effectiveness and Efficiency

Edited by
Andrew F. Long and Stephen Harrison

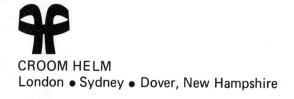

CROOM HELM
London • Sydney • Dover, New Hampshire

Croom Helm Ltd, Provident House, Burrell Row,
Beckenham, Kent BR3 1AT

Croom Helm Australia Pty Ltd, First Floor,
139 King Street, Sydney, NSW 2001, Australia

British Library Cataloguing in Publication Data

Health service performance : effectiveness and
   efficiency.
   1. Medical care – Evaluation
   I. Long, A.F. II. Harrison, Stephen
   362.1   RA399.A1

   ISBN 0-7099-1672-8

Croom Helm, 51 Washington Street, Dover,
New Hampshire 03820,USA

Library of Congress Cataloging in Publication Data
Main entry under title:

Health services performance.

   Bibliography: p.
   Includes index
   1. Medical care – Evaluation – Addresses, Essays,
Lectures. 2. Medical Care – Quality Control – Addresses,
Essays, Lectures. 3. Medical Care – Cost Effectiveness –
Addresses, Essays, Lectures. I. Long, A.F. (Andrew F.)
II. Harrison, Stephen, 1947- . (DNLM: 1. Health
Services – Organization & Administration. 2. Quality
Assurance, Health Care. W 84.1 H4378)
RA399.A1H43   1985   362.1   85-1310
ISBN 0-7099-1672-8

Printed and bound in Great Britain by
Biddles Ltd, Guildford and King's Lynn

CONTENTS

TABLES

Tables

FIGURES

ACKNOWLEDGEMENTS

We acknowledge the helpful comments of Andrew Green on parts of this text. Most importantly, however, we thank Carole Munro for typing the several drafts, and preparing the final manuscript of this book for publication.

The views expressed in this volume are those of the contributors as individuals and not necessarily those of their parent organisation.

Finally in our role as editors we are grateful to our fellow contributors for their hard work and cooperation in this project.

ANDREW F LONG
STEPHEN HARRISON

Chapter 1

HEALTH SERVICES PERFORMANCE: AN OVERVIEW

Andrew F. Long and Stephen Harrison

Although it has been recognised for more than twenty
years that the demand for health care is potentially
unlimited, whereas resources are not, attempts to
face this dilemma have until recent years
concentrated on organisational, rather than
behavioural, solutions. In the past five years
however, the failure of such strategy, coupled with
the deepening of an economic recession, has led to
more specific attempts to contain the costs of
health services delivery, in particular through the
exploration of ways to define, measure, and improve
the performance of health service organisations.
    Such a scenario relates easily to the health
care systems of Europe and North America, three of
which countries are explored in this volume of
essays: Britain, Canada, and the United States of
America. In Britain, attention has in the last five
years centred on the notion of performance review,
coupled with strict financial controls on resource
input (cash limits and manpower targets), and sets
of performance indicators oriented towards the
search for value for money and accountability (Klein
1982). In the USA and Canada, the search for
efficiency and quality assurance has similarly been
extensively waged, but with greater intensity in
recent years.
    Many questions are raised by such developments.
Firstly, why is there this relatively sudden
manifestation of concern with controlling costs?
There are many candidates for explanation, including
the general world economic situation, the growing
orthodoxy of monetarist economics, the ideological
suspicion of conservative politicians for all forms
of state expenditure, the growing numbers and
assertiveness of the different groups of actors
involved in the production and consumption of health

1

care, and the growing intellectual critiques of modern medicine by sociologists, economists and epidemiologists. Secondly, is the concern simply with the lowest common denominator of total health care costs, or with some more sophisticated notion of 'performance'? Thirdly, what kinds of policy result from this general concern, how are they implemented, and what are the results?

It is to the exploration of these and other related issues that this volume of essays is directed. As a preliminary to such an investigation it is important though to elucidate briefly what the concepts of 'performance' and 'quality assurance' entail. This is the subject of the remainder of this introductory Chapter, together with an overview of the other essays in this volume.

PERFORMANCE, QUALITY ASSURANCE AND EVALUATION

The notions of performance and quality assurance, and associated mechanisms for exploring and applying them, describe the activity of evaluating health care services. Holland (1983 p. 8) defines the process of evaluation as '... the formal determination of the effectiveness, efficiency, and acceptability of a planned intervention in achieving stated objectives.' Effectiveness can then be defined as a measure of the technical outcome of health services, in medical, social and/or psychological terms, efficiency as the ratio of the product produced to resource input, and acceptability as the judgement of an intervention as professionally and/or socially satisfactory and adequate. In this vein, performance review and quality assurance are means to the end of evaluating (health care) services with a view to their effectiveness, efficiency and acceptability. The discussions in Chapters 2, 3, and 4 respectively examine these aspects in detail.

The process of evaluation can further be usefully subdivided into two aspects: quality assessment and quality assurance. (Donabedian 1966 and 1980) In the quality assessment phase, attention is upon the measurement of the level of quality of services provided, involving a concern with defining what is to be evaluated, the development of indicators of measurement, and the generation of monitoring data systems. The second phase encompasses the use of the monitoring indices, with a view to assessing the current quality of service provided, and the generation where necessary of efforts to modify existing service provision in the light of the indicators of performance. Attention shifts from the measurement process itself to mechanisms of control and the political nexus surrounding the provision of services.

The comments of Luke and Boss (1981 p. 305) are apposite here on what they see as three major barriers to quality assurance: '... the conceptualisation, the measurement, and the assessment. The major conceptual barrier is simply to determine what quality is.' The question of 'from whose perspective?' can usefully be added. But, they continue, once a satisfactory definition of quality is identified, the second barrier of measurement is faced. There is also the difficulty of selecting an appropriate assessment strategy. Even if all these problems and difficulties are surmounted, 'the real question is not whether such technical problems can be resolved, but whether it is appropriate to assume that providing people or organisations with data will change their behaviour.' (Luke and Boss 1981 p. 306) Thus the implementation aspect comes finally to the fore.

Luke and Boss's first question of the definition of quality can be approached by reference to the work of Vuori (1982). He discusses four issues: effectiveness, efficiency, equity and quality. Firstly, he argues, a service has to be capable of producing the desired effects in terms of the provision of health care to patients. It must be capable (in theory) and do so in practice. The concept of effectiveness describes this concern, that is, the relationship of the actual to the potential impact in an ideal organisational and environmental setting. Secondly, the service must be produced efficiently, at an optimal cost. Thirdly, it must be provided according to the principle of equity in its distribution, in relation to the perceived health needs of the population. Again the question of 'from whose perspective' can be raised, such variations in perception potentially leading to perceptions of inequity. Fourthly, the service must adhere to the fundamental principle of quality: that is, applying currently available medical knowledge and technology in an ethical manner within a given set of structural (manpower, finance, and available technical equipment) constraints.

Such a set of principles provides a baseline for evaluating health services. They also raise

several prerequisites for any successful attempt at
reviewing services. Firstly, it is essential to
understand the cause and effect relationship between
resource use and the process of care provided and
any health status outcome. Without such knowledge,
no comment can be made on the effectiveness of the
health care service. Closely allied to this
issue is the second prerequisite of an extensive
and relevant information base. This involves the
prior stage of identifying measures of health
services performance on the three axes of
effectiveness, efficiency and acceptability. In
many examples of measures of performance, the
information system used takes no account of health
outcomes. To be a satisfactory indicator of
performance, two conditions have to be met: firstly,
the treatment or activity is generally acknowledged
to be effective for the particular disorder in
question; and secondly, treatment is only applied to
those who will benefit from it. (Lewis and Modle
1982 p. 4)

A third prerequisite, and perhaps the most
critical of all, is the organisational, personal,
and societal commitment to both the principles of
and the need for quality assurance. In this
respect, the environment in which performance review
occurs cannot be ignored. The factors influencing
the health system including revenue, indicated
governmental priorities and societal expectations
of services, and the factors determining health
itself and the contribution health services can make
in theory and in practice to the level of health of
the population and in caring for the ill, all
influence the level of commitment to the evaluation
process. There is too the environment of the
quality assurance process itself: that is, the
legal, political, professional and social values,
norms and attitudes governing it. (Vuori 1982)
Donabedian's (1980) differentiation between the
'technical' and the 'interpersonal' aspects of
quality is relevant here. The technical aspect
involves the application of medical science and
technology to maximise the benefit to health without
a corresponding increase in its risks. The
interpersonal aspect relates to the need for the
quality of services to meet socially defined norms
and values, reinforced by the ethics of health
practitioners, and the expectations of patients.
The two aspects are clearly closely interrelated.
The environment can thus detract from the assurance
of quality or positively provide support and

commitment.

Without such a commitment, not only can the results of the performance review not be implemented, but also little effort will go into generating sound monitoring tools. Commitment, it is argued, must be placed not on just one of the elements of the process, be it effectiveness, efficiency, or acceptability, but on them all. Otherwise it is easy to imagine a situation where a health service may be highly efficient, yet providing ineffective and unacceptable care to the consumer. Commitment to an effective, efficient and acceptable service must be the aim. The fact that, as Vuori (1982 p. 80) points out, these three issues are potentially contradictory in terms of the goals of the funders, the providers and the consumers must not be minimised or ignored. In the design of a quality assurance or performance review programme, the issue of the multiplicity of perspectives on acceptability and effectiveness must be addressed and reasons given explicitly for choices made. Whether or not such prerequisites are met in practice, and whether the consumer's view in addition to that of the health services providers' is taken into account is a topic which many of the Chapters in this volume explore.

Discussion so far has highlighted a number of issues. Firstly, the performance of a health service must be viewed in relation to three aspects: its effectiveness, its efficiency, and its acceptability. Each of these concepts in turn requires detailed elaboration, a task addressed in the first four Chapters of this book. Secondly, the need for good information systems was identified, as well as knowledge of the link between the input of health services and output in terms of patient health status outcomes. Thirdly, the varying perspectives of the three sets of actors in health services (health care funders, practitioners and consumers) in relation to performance, and in particular in relation to effectiveness and acceptability ('who is to define quality?') was raised. Evaluation is by definition a value-laden activity, and must be acknowledged to be so, thus suggesting the need to take all relevant parties' views into consideration. Finally, the issue of implementation and in particular the level of commitment to performance review is raised and explored in detail in Chapter 5. One issue outstanding is the question of the performance or quality of 'what?'.

Donabedian (1980) argues that the evaluation of the quality of care (and health services) involves the functional relationship of structure - process - outcome. That is, the structural characteristics of settings affect the process of care which affects the outcome of that care. None of these three, he argues, represent attributes of quality, but each provides an approach to generating information on the presence or absence of quality. Thus, in principle, performance can be evaluated by looking at any of these three aspects. Indeed, it is often conceptually easier to look at structure and process than at outcome. This leads to the danger of making over-simplistic assumptions about the relationship between these two and outcome.

Assessing the 'structure' of care is thus one option in assessing performance. 'Structure is relevant to quality in that it increases or decreases the probability of good performance.' (Donabedian 1980 p. 82) It is then only a facilitator, and most importantly a means for acting on the findings of the quality of services. It thus provides a blunt instrument to assess quality, having an unclear link to performance. An additional problem is that of the stability of the structure over time.

Assessing the 'outcome' is similarly problematic. Concern lies with the change in the patient's current and/or future health state and its attribution to antecedent health care. Leaving aside the problem of the measurement of health and the need to address not only the health practitioner's perception but also that of the patient, there remains the difficulty of ascertaining with any degree of certainty that the change in health status was caused by the preceding health care. Only once one knows that a particular process of care leads to certain results can one accept that the mere presence (or absence) of such processes is evidence of good (or bad) quality. Furthermore, as Donabedian points out, if changes in health status are observed, then not only must there be a prior basis for assuming a possible relationship (the issue of causal validity), but also one must show that other possible (causal) factors are absent (the issue of attributional validity), which might otherwise explain the change in health status. This issue is further explored in Chapter 2 of this volume.

Finally, assessment of the 'process' of care is not without its limitations. For while health care practitioners may have little difficulty in identifying facets and standards of good practice, and the actual management of the patient tends to be reasonably well documented in the patient's medical record, norms and standards of practice have a weak scientific basis. (Donabedian 1980 p. 119) In the USA, the shadow of negligence and physician liability looms over medical practice, with a resultant tendency towards elaborate and costly care. There is too the issue of the interpersonal aspect of quality; where does this fit into the assessment of quality through a process approach? Is it ethical for the physicians to take over the rights of the patient and judge what is appropriate? (Miesel 1981) In contrast to this overemphasis on technical care, the management of the interpersonal process tends to be ignored, partly because the criteria represent primarily the practitioner's concerns and partly because the usual sources of data give little information about the practitioner-patient relationship. (Donabedian 1980 p. 119)

Utilising Donabedian's functional relationship of structure, process and outcome, it becomes apparent that assessing quality cannot be adequately undertaken by looking at one element alone. All three are intimately related. Donabedian points out that an important advantage of outcome evaluation is that it '... tends to discourage dogmatism ... (and that) outcomes reflect all the contributions of all the practitioners to the care of the patient, ... (providing) an inclusive integrative measure of the quality of care.' (1980 p. 120) It also allows the possibility of taking the consumer's own perspective (client satisfaction) into account. But there are too the issues of causal and attributional validity. Any system of assessing quality must thus address all three aspects, a similar conclusion to that drawn earlier in relation to the three components of evaluation of health care services. A system of performance review addressing all the three aspects of effectiveness, efficiency, and acceptability must be the aim, taking into account not only the health practitioners' but also the health consumers' perspectives.

OVERVIEW OF THE BOOK

Building on this elaboration of the dimensions and problems in defining performance and quality, the following three Chapters of this book explore the three main aspects of performance. Accordingly, Chapter 2 examines the concept of effectiveness and its definition. It argues that the main thrust of assessing performance must lie on examining the relationship between health care needs and health status outcomes. Accordingly, attention centres on identifying determinants of health and the potential contributions of the health services to reducing the level of illness in the community, in addition to its caring role, and on examining possible measures of health to employ as measures of outcome. The need to take into account the consumer's own perceptions in addition to those of the health practitioner is strongly argued for. The final section of the Chapter presents a series of evaluative questions to assist in reviewing research on the effectiveness of health service programme or intervention, and of current services provided.

In Chapter 3 attention centres on the notion of efficiency, and explores its various aspects: allocative, distributive, managerial and dynamic efficiency. In so doing, issues of measurement and data sources and their relationship to financial management practices are examined. The Chapter ends with a summary of the major differences of approach to efficiency, and contrasts the economist's and the accountant's perspective.

Chapter 4 picks up the remaining aspect of evaluation, namely acceptability. From the definition of acceptability, the first issue to address is that of 'acceptable to whom?' and 'from whose perspective?'. The Chapter accordingly examines acceptability from the viewpoint of health care producers and consumers. A case study of one Regional Health Authority is presented highlighting the complexity of the situation and the relative voices of the interested parties.

Discussion in Chapter 5 turns to what has earlier been described as a critical element in the whole process of performance review/quality assurance: that is, the issue of implementation. Theoretical approaches to actors' perceptions and actions are reviewed and an attempt made to identify empirical evidence in support of each. No one theoretical view is seen as adequately explaining the situation. The Chapter uses a range of such views to pose a number of fundamental questions about the process of evaluating health services performance.

Chapter 5 also serves to link together the theoretical and definitional nature of the previous three Chapters to the review of attention given and approaches employed in the area of performance and quality assurance in Britain (Chapter 6), the Canada (Chapter 7), and the United States of America (Chapter 8). Each of these Chapters aims to explore the actual application and consideration given to the notions of effectiveness, efficiency, and acceptability, and to examine the way performance review is approached and implemented.

The final Chapter attempts to draw together the empirical material from the three countries reviewed and the theory identified in earlier Chapters. Discussion centres around three questions in an attempt to clarify some of the choices and issues which underlie discussion about health services: the origins of a concern with performance, the definition and perception of performance, and problems of implementations. The Chapter closes by examining the implications of current approaches to health services performance, and argues for the pursuit of a broad approach to performance embracing the three aspects of effectiveness, efficiency, and acceptability.

Chapter 2

EFFECTIVENESS: DEFINITIONS AND APPROACHES

Andrew F. Long

'A physician who tries a remedy and cures his
patients is inclined to believe that the cure is due
to his treatment. Physicians often pride themselves
on curing all their patients with a remedy they use.
But the first thing to ask them is whether they have
tried doing nothing, that is not treating
other patients; for how can they otherwise know
whether the remedy or nature cured them.' (Bernard
1927 p. 194)
     This observation was made by Claude Bernard, a
distinguished French physician (1865-1949),
advocating to his medical colleagues the need for
evaluation of their current and proposed practice
in terms of its effectiveness. In his own work, he
pioneered such research using the approach of a
comparison group and randomisation to ensure valid
conclusions. His comment is as relevant now as
then, and has been taken up by many commentators
since. (Cochrane 1972; Illsley 1980)
Problematically, however, once a particular
technique or therapy is found to be the 'most'
effective of those available (leaving aside the
notion of cost for the moment), the issue of
effectiveness is not solved for all time. Potential
modifications in treatment and medical practice,
developments in drug therapy, knowledge of the
causes of the illness (raising the possibility of
primary preventive action), and emerging
technologies will necessitate a continuing
evaluative approach. At first 'no' treatment must
be compared with a treatment, and if the treatment
is then deemed 'more' effective, the 'old' treatment
will be contrasted with the 'new', prior to the
general introduction of the replacement therapy. In
this way, Bernard's advice is not only sound but
relevant to current concerns over health services

performance.
　　This Chapter does not however seek to review current, or potential, medical and more general health services practice with a view to the effectiveness of treatment generally or interventions for specific illnesses. Its intention is more fundamental: to examine definitions and approaches to the very notion of effectiveness in the context of health services provision. Discussion is divided into three parts. First of all, the general meaning of the concept 'effectiveness' is examined, and several extensions to the simple definition explored. It is argued that the basic dimension of debate should centre on the relationship, and any mismatch, between health 'needs' and health 'outcome'. Such an approach inevitably raises problems of application which is the focus of the second part of the Chapter. In particular, potential measures of health outcome are reviewed, together with a discussion of strategies to assess the effectiveness of a service, health programme or intervention, issues surrounding the imputation of causality (what are the causes of illness, and will the health services programme have any, let alone the desired, effect?), and aspects of data requirements and sources. In the third section, a checklist of questions to assist in reviewing the effectiveness of a service is drawn up. The objective of the Chapter is thus to clarify the notion of effectiveness, as well as to point towards approaches to its exploration and potential achievement.

DEFINITIONS AND APPROACHES TO EFFECTIVENESS

As a general starting point, the concept of effectiveness in health services performance can be defined as a measure of the degree to which the objective(s) of a policy programme, treatment, pattern of care, or resource group has been achieved. The critical feature of such a definition is the explicit link of the objectives of the service or procedure to actual performance: that is the achievement of the objectives. Effectiveness is thus bound up with the production of a desired effect, in contrast to efficiency (the subject of Chapter Three) the focus of which lies on the achievement of the maximal result with minimum effort or inputs.
　　Such a definition throws into sharp relief four

stages for exploring the effectiveness of health service practice. (Vuori 1982; Holland 1983) The initial stage is to identify the objectives set for the service, manpower group or programme itself: that is, the baseline of 'minimum', 'better', or 'best' care. If no objectives have been set, no assessment of effectiveness can be made. The very concept of effectiveness becomes meaningless unless clear objectives are identified and set in the establishment of a service or programme. This point can be taken a step further and the case argued that the objectives must be stated in a quantitative manner, or at a minimum in a manner amenable to measurement. For otherwise it remains a matter of debate of whether the objectives have been met or not. This leads straightforwardly to the second stage, consisting of drawing up an indicator or set of indicators which can measure the degree to which the objectives are being met. Problems of data sources, and of defining and measuring the objectives in a reliable and valid manner are paramount here. The third stage is that of comparing the outcome of the programme with the desired end-state. Any shortfall can then be identified and explanatory reasons postulated. The final stage is aimed at exploring ways to maximise the achievement of the programme's objectives, thus modifying the service or programme or pattern of delivery. It must be noted that one simple and obvious way to ensure an effective service, under this definition, is to lower the objectives or targets of the programme to make them achievable. Furthermore, objectives of a health programme and its direction towards a particular target population may be modified by features of access to the programme because of inequitable distribution, income constraints, historical usage patterns, or patients' expectations and beliefs regarding appropriate health care services.

This general definition can with benefit be made more specific without losing the essential feature of a link between an objective and its achievement. Holland (1983 p. 274), with an eye to the epidemiological use of the term 'effectiveness', defines it as '... a measure of the degree to which a particular treatment or pattern of care in the population achieves its objective in medical, psychological, and social terms.' In other words, has the state of health of individuals in the population increased as a result of a health service programme, or a deterioration been avoided that would otherwise have occurred? Once so specified, it becomes more difficult to sidestep the essential nature of the concept of effectiveness, and also more important to state the objectives in such a manner as to be amenable to translation into quantitative targets. It should be noted that such an extension to the definition can easily be amended to apply to the clinician's field of activity, that is, to refer to the effectiveness of an episide of care for a particular patient. Such a clinical viewpoint is however outside the frame of reference of this Chapter, where the focus is epidemiological, addressing the effectiveness of health services, or the effectiveness of a particular programme of clinical care for a group of patients or a wider community.

Building on this basic definition, Holland (1983) differentiates four aspects of effectiveness. Firstly, there is 'population effectiveness': that is, the ability of a health service (medical) intervention to produce a measurable improvement in the health of the population as a whole. Closely allied is the concept of 'attributable effectiveness' defined as the difference between the outcome in a group exposed to a health care programme or treatment and a group given a different (or no) treatment. The concern is to show the extent to which the change in health status in the patients resulted from the treatment programme. Thirdly, there is 'population attributable effectiveness': the number of persons within a population who would gain from receiving a health care programme. This is a measure of the 'impact' of the programme on the population. It is in this way that Vuori (1982 p. 37) defines effectiveness: as '... the relation of the actual impact of a service or programme in an operating system to its full potential impact in an ideal situation.' Finally, there is 'relative effectiveness': the ratio of the outcome between individuals receiving a health care programme and those who are not.

These several specifications of the concept of effectiveness point towards the possibility of employing a variety of approaches in exploring the effectiveness of a health care programme or procedure. A possible ordering of these several definitions in terms of their use in reviewing the effectivnesss of a service is as follows. Firstly, attention would centre on establishing whether a programme leads to changes in the health status of the target population. This requires an emphasis on population effectiveness. At the same time, as a necessary consequence, focus would lie on seeing whether the change was brought about by the programme or something else which is likely to be unspecified. This involves an emphasis on attributable effectiveness. Secondly, the relative benefits of one programme versus another would be addressed, and/or the degree to which the change in health status was brought about by the programme. This is an emphasis on relative effectiveness. Finally, the degree of impact on the target population if the programme were to be made available would be identified. The emphasis eventually lies on population attributable effectiveness, that is, the programme's impact on the target population, the undoubted aim of any intervention or procedure. Once the chain of effectiveness has been established concern will then need to shift towards the economist's viewpoint of '... maximising the difference between total social benefits and total social costs.' (Williams 1974 p. 196)

The economist's approaches to economic appraisal, namely the techniques of cost-benefit (CBA) and cost-effectiveness analysis (CEA), are highly germane at this point, as they relate respectively to the general notion of effectiveness and relative effectiveness. In CBA, the objectives of a programme or health intervention can be questioned. The very desirability of the programme in the long and the short term is addressed focussing on potential side effects, social benefits and opportunity costs. CEA, on the other hand, takes the objectives as they are and attempts to ascertain how to achieve them at a minimum cost. It either addresses the issue of which of a set of equally costly alternatives is most effective, or which of several equally effective treatments is less costly. (Drummond 1980)

As a final contribution to this discussion concerning the definition of effectiveness it is valuable to look at the implied definition given by Donabedian (1980) in his exploration of the concept of the quality of care. Quality of care, he argues, has two components. Firstly, there is the technical component, which involves the application of medical science and technology to maximise the benefit without correspondingly increasing the risk to the patient's health. Secondly, there is an inter-personal dimension to quality, involving the management of the social and psychological interaction between the patient and the health practitioner. Care in this sense must meet socially defined values and norms: the notion of acceptabilty discussed in Chapter Four of this volume. So, quality becomes '... the kind of care that maximises an inclusive measure of patient welfare.' (Donabedian 1980 p. 6) But such quality may be expensive. In any definition and approach to effectiveness then, the link between the health gains and risks attached to a health care programme must be explored, as must the health gain-risk balance and costs (financial, social and others) of a programme.

The concept of effectiveness links objectives to their achievement. Such objectives will have to be defined in relation to notions of equity and perceived health need. In this way, effectiveness would seem to centre on the relationship between the health 'needs' of the population and any outcomes following a health (and non-health) services intervention, and any mismatch between needs and outcome. A range of perspectives in defining and measuring health needs exists, finding correspondence in similar diversity in terms of the defining perspective for effectiveness. For, should focus lie on the individual consumer's viewpoint, or the health practitioner's or a wider societal view, or should it be a combination of the three? If the health practitioner's viewpoint is dominant and the patient's needs are predetermined, there remains the difficulty of getting consumers to come forward for the service, even if a screening programme is designed. In other words, it is the potential patients who 'demand' and use health services. Similar comments apply to approaches to assessing effectiveness, and in particular to whether or not the consumer's view of services should be taken into account.

Building on this needs-outcome dimension, a number of points can be made. Firstly, it is clear that the health services themselves are not the only, nor necessarily the most important factor in determining health outcomes. There are other major features of society which affect health, for example, housing, water and sewage disposal, and general affluence. (McKeown 1976; Townsend and Davidson 1982) Spontaneous recoveries from episodes of ill health also occur. This point will be discussed further below in exploring the determinants of health and illness. Secondly, in identifying the actual contribution of a particular health intervention to health status (a population and attributable effectiveness concern), research tends to focus on a relevant high-risk sub-group: for example, the heavy smokers with a poor diet in a preventive programme on coronary heart disease. Once it is shown that the intervention is effective (in reducing the incidence of heart disease, following a reduction in the intervened risk indicators), then the question arises as to whether to broaden the programme for others at lower risk and to identify what impact it will have: that is, can one generalise from these research subjects to a lower risk group? The logical conclusion is that of 'not really', which finds backing in relevant research. (Oliver 1983; Stallones 1983)

This simple depiction of effectiveness as being concerned with matching needs and outcomes points to two other major issues. Firstly, there is the question of how to measure need, and outcomes, and from whose perspective. In epidemiological terms, the key issue becomes one of identifying relevant populations (McCarthy 1982a) and defining the 'need for a (health or health related) service.' Some possible approaches are explored below. Secondly, objectives indicating desired health outcomes are essential in monitoring the activity and direction of the health services. As McCarthy (1982a and 1982b) argues, it becomes of paramount importance to set 'outcome targets', which themselves must be based on sound epidemiological research findings.

The discussion so far has examined several approaches to the definition of the concept of effectiveness in the context of health service performance evaluation. The basic concept has been described as one involving the connection between the objective of a health care programme and the actual performance of the programme, and more succinctly as the (mis)match between needs and outcomes. Once the objective of a programme is stated, attention can centre on the effectiveness of its achievement. In terms of health care the objectives of an intervention will inevitably have to be stated in relation to changes in the health status of the consumers of the programme (outcome targets). Several fundamental problems were pointed out: namely, how are health status need and outcome to be defined and then measured? whose perspective of health and by implication of the quality of care will be employed – the consumers', the health practitioners' or the policy-makers'? where and how

can data on individuals' health status be obtained?
and how can one be sure that the changes in health
status observed were actually brought about by the
health care programme? It is to a consideration
of these questions that the discussion now turns.

DEFINING HEALTH, NEED, AND OUTCOME

Effectiveness as defined above relates to the
achievement of the objectives of a health care
programme, which it was suggested will be phrased in
terms of changes in health status among its
recipients. In this regard it becomes of paramount
importance to explore the various meanings and
perspectives of health status and need, to identify
ways of measuring them, and to develop, as
appropriate, data sources to monitor any changes in
health status. However it should be noted that the
objective of a programme does not always have to be
stated in terms of changes in health status, or the
relationship of need to outcome. This will only be
the case where interest lies in outcome evaluation.
For, all outcome studies address the issue of the
value of a programme or intervention in the effect
it has on the recipients' state of health. But in
the context of an evaluation of the process of care
this is unlikely to be the case, except in a
secondary manner where a direct link to a health
outcome is suggested. Sound objectives for a
process evaluation could be ones relating to
increasing the throughput in a unit, reducing the
length of stay, or identifying the appropriate
place or form of treatment for a condition. Such
objectives of course focus on the efficiency of the
health programme at the forefront of their
attention. But, in assessing the achievement of the
objectives, effectiveness is also their concern. In
this regard, Vuori (1982 p. 82) distinguishes
between a 'process outcome' (such as the number of
examinations performed or the throughput of a unit),
and a 'product outcome' (changes in the health
states of a target population). Only the latter, he
argues has a clear link back to the objectives of
the programme. Furthermore, if there is no clear
objective, then exploring process outcomes is the
next best thing. This has perhaps served to
underline the terminological difficulties that
abound in the area, unless effectiveness is
specifically linked to a concern with changes in
health for a target population, and the relationship

of need and health outcome.

The notion of health has been extensively discussed in the literature. [1] Accordingly, only a brief review of some of the major issues will be provided in order to illuminate options for the measurement of health, so essential to an evaluation of the effectiveness of a service. Definitions of health involve reference to the concept of normality; health is normal and ill-health abnormal. Such a statement is a little simplistic. Empirically, few people at any one time have any one illness, such as lung cancer, cirrhosis of the liver, or heart disease. At the same time, many people may not say that they are' well', in the sense of 'totally fit', or without any ache, pain, or anxiety. The question of healthy 'from whose perspective' arises again. If clinical definitions are employed, statistics of health utilisation point to large numbers of episodes of ill-health; and if investigations of clinically perceived need are followed, more illness will no doubt be uncovered. Furthermore, once attention turns to the individual's self perception of health and illness, given health's position as a highly valued state, indeed as a desideratum, perfect health becomes an unlikely finding. [2] As Antonovsky (1980) observed, the more one probes, the more the individual respondent is likely to identify a symptom or feeling of malaise. Wadsworth's (1971) finding in Great Britain that 5% of his 2000 or so respondents perceived themselves as healthy, and 95% as not or were currently under some form of medical care, is thus unsurprising.

Any statement and measure of health is thus based on a value judgement, itself founded on the premise that health is an ideal – the positive health notion expounded by the World Health Organisation, as meaning not merely the absence of disease and disability, but complete mental, physical, and social well-being. There is too the confounding factor that health may be differently perceived and defined by health practitioners and lay people. This applies not only to perspectives of health, but also of need. For example, Holland (1983 p. 68) draws up a typology composed of the three elements of medically defined need for health care, socially defined need, and individually perceived need (Figure 2.1). He observes that the aim of health services is at least to meet medically defined need, and thus to also take into account social and individual perceptions. [3] In only two

instances do all the three definitions concur on the
need or non-need for health care. In addition there
is the complication of the demand (the translation
of perceived need into action) and utilisation
(involving the concepts of access and equity) of
health services and their relationship to need. It
remains a matter of empirical research as to the
actual mismatch between the various perspectives,
but the potential for confusion remains. Whose
perspective to employ is an issue that cannot be
ignored.

Taking this discussion a step further, it is
valuable to refer to the conceptualisation of health
expounded by Susser (1974). Health is viewed on
three dimensions (Table 2.1). Firstly, there is the
organic, physiological dimension which is defined by
medical science and technology and diagnosed and
perceived by health practitioners. Secondly, there
is the functional dimension, relating to the
individual's own viewpoint on health (his/her self-
perception). Thirdly, there is a more general
societal view, referring to socially recognised or
acknowledged limitations of an individual's role
(for example, in the normal activities of daily
living), often to be legitimated by health
practitioners. So, not only can health be defined
and perceived differently by the several key actors
(health practitioners, consumers, and policy
makers), but also different dimensions may even be
addressed. The similarity of this conceptualisation
to Holland's model of need can be noted too. As
Susser points out, perceptions of health may vary
over time, and one dimension may expand and tend to
predominate. Currently, in industrialised
countries, medicine focusses on the organic level
(to identify and cure disease, as well as to care
for the terminally ill), and also on the social
level (to rationalise and legitimate illness).
Identifying and maintaining a balance in perspective
may then be the major issue, or even as in the
British NHS (in contrast to the USA) the need to
pay more heed to the consumer's view, and their
'right to know' about potential treatments or health
programmes, and their effectiveness.

The above remarks have stressed that the
definition of health need and outcome varies
according to who is defining it and which aspect has
priority. The situation is compounded by variations
in access to health services, in tolerance of pain
and discomfort, and in attitudes to and expectations
of health services. Lay people's perceptions of

Figure 2.1: Typology of Need for Health Services

		Medically Defined Need			
		No		Yes	
		Socially determined need		Socially determined need	
		No	Yes	No	Yes
Perceived Need	No	No need	Medically unjustified social need without perceived need	Hidden medically defined need only	Medical and social need without perceived need
	Yes	Unjustifed perceived need	Medically unjustified perceived and social need	Medical and perceived need without behavioural disturbances	Unanimous need

Source: Holland, 1983, p. 68

Table 2.1: Three Dimensions of Health (Susser 1974)

DIMENSION	DEFINED BY
1. ORGANIC/PHYSIOLOGICAL	(MEDICS)

1. ORGANIC/PHYSIOLOGICAL   (MEDICS)
   Changes in organism, in physiology - the
   signs and symptoms of Disease or their long-term
   consequences resulting in Impairment.

2. FUNCTIONAL   (INDIVIDUALS)
   Individual's subjective state of psychological
   awareness of ill-health, or limitations in
   functioning - Illness, or if a long-term
   limitation in functioning Disability.

3. SOCIAL   (MEDICS)
                                               ('SOCIETY')
   Limitations in performing one's role in society;
   socially accepted limitations, or socially
   acknowledged - Sickness, or if long term,
   Handicap.

what constitutes illness, of the relevance of health
services (Mechanic 1962; Dingwall 1976) become
important factors to take into consideration. The
dominant paradigm over definitions of health and
need is medical, where the health practitioner
diagnoses disease on the basis of signs and
symptoms, backed up by medical technology, and
incomplete knowledge of the physiological effects of
disease and their causes. A patient is diseased or
not, or else a malingerer or a hypochondriac.
Antonovsky (1980) describes this as the pathogenic
model of disease. Physiological variations are the
focus, to the detriment of the functional dimension
of health. The patient's perceptions are taken into
account only in that they guide the initial decision
over whether to make use of health services. Once
such a decision is made the 'science of disease' is
appealed to, and health care then falls largely out
of the patient's hands. It must be pointed out that
the physician in a complicated manner gives
attention to the social dimension of illness, in his
role as the legitimator of illness. (Freidson 1970)
What constitutes legitimate illness from the
perspective of society relates back to the role of
political and economic ideology within the society.
The individual's own perception of what is wrong, or

21

his/her need, or valuation of the outcome of health
care is accorded low significance in contrast to
clinically defined need. The result of a
biochemical test or a scan becomes of greater
importance than the patient's own feelings and
perceptions.
        Whose perspective on health should be adopted
within an evaluation of the effectiveness of a
health programme? There are three options.
Firstly, there is the definition of the health
practitioners and the providers of the service. The
likely definitions of health and need will be ones
relating to the medical perspective, given their
dominant position within the health organisation,
and the professionalisation of medicine and health
care. (Freidson 1970; Larkin 1983) The very
structure and composition of the health programme
will then be seen in terms of clinically defined
need and changes in health status in relation to the
current state of knowledge on the causes of the
illness under focus and the art of implementation of
the treatment regime. Secondly, there is the
definition of the prospective user of the service.
At least to some extent their viewpoint will have to
be taken into account; for if an alternative to the
service exists the individual may not make use of
the programme. However, as Donabedian (1980)
comments, the health service cannot be directed at
each individual's viewpoint; it must rather create
criteria and standards applicable to the many. This
then leads to the third option, of addressing a
social definition, in which to the individual view
is appended the criterion of 'aggregate net benefit
or utility' for the population as a whole. This
leaves open the possibility of giving greater
weight to deprived sections of the community, a
view strongly argued by Morris (1982). One can
thus conclude that while traditionally the
quality of care has focussed on the physiological
dimension of health, should it not now be expanded
to take into account a broader definition of
health, and in particular the perspective of the
lay person? Both Donabedian (1980) and Vuori
(1982) concur in this regard; it is the community's
valuation of states of health, of indicators of
provision, that are important, and must then
be addressed in identifying need, measuring
health outcome, and in expressing the
effectiveness of a health programme.
        The issue is clearly not one of either-or, but
of identifying a relevant measure of health for the

particular health programme or intervention under review. For example, a programme aimed at reducing the incidence of an illness could with benefit take into account the functional, the organic and the social dimensions of health. Focus could lie on the incidence of the illness, its effect is on the ability to perform activities of daily living, and the consequences of any handicaps. There is, too, the issue of who has the responsibility for ensuring that the service is effective. The terms in which effectiveness is to be judged may then be weighted in their favour. In this connection Vuori's (1982 p. 9-11) comments on the interest profile of sponsoring agencies for quality assurance is of interest. He puts forward the proposition that effectiveness is of high concern to the consumers of health services and only to a limited extent to the health practitioners, and of virtually no interest to health authorities (local and central agencies). For the health practitioners the main issue is one of quality, that is, providing the best care available given current medical knowledge and technology; and for the health authorities, their main interest lies in efficiency. In conclusion, whatever position is adopted it is important to make clear that a choice over whose perspective in defining health and need has been made; furthermore, reasons should be indicated to support the position adopted, and to make it plain why the emphasis lies there. The consumer or layperson's perspective, in terms of a 'right to know' and 'satisfaction' with the health service, must not be left off the agenda.

POTENTIAL MEASURES OF HEALTH OUTCOME

Several measures of health have been put forward in the literature which would seem to have promise in relation to explorations of the effectiveness of health care services. In particular there are the approaches of Rutstein et al (1976) and subsequently Charlton et al (1983); Rosser and Watts (1972) and Fanshel (1972); and attempts to develop general measures of health such as the Nottingham health profile (Hunt et al 1980, 1984) and Antonovsky's breakdown concept (1973, 1980). These are only a few among the many. The intention is to review some of their features, in order to gain insight into possible ways for measuring health for use in studies of effectiveness.

As a starting point it is valuable to look at the definition and measurement of health implied in current studies in the field, and to point to some of their difficulties. It is not surprising, given earlier remarks, to find that effectiveness studies have tended to be undertaken from within the pathogenic model. In trying to identify suitable measures of health resort has been made to the 'spectrum model of disease' widely employed in epidemiology (Figure 2.2). Accordingly, focus will fall on the effect of a health programme on the natural history of disease, and in particular the ability either to prevent death from a specific cause or to reduce the probability of such death through the means of earlier diagnosis, better treatment or, more rarely, attempts to eradicate the cause from the environment of the community (primary prevention). However, while this approach is eminently sound in principle, the chosen measure to assess effectiveness has become that of mortality: for example, comparisons of case fatality rates resulting from alternative forms of treatment, or perinatal and infant mortality rates, standardised for birth weight and the age of the mother, or the use of survival analysis leading to figures on the expectation of life to evaluate two or more treatments.

While the assessment of differences in mortality rates is simple and the relevant data are easily available and no measuremnt problems exist, this approach is not without its drawbacks. In the case of life-threatening diseases, death, survival or cure may provide adequate, if not good, outcomes (achievements) of health care. (Holland 1983) For other situations, it is not so straightforward. Firstly, once interest starts to fall on the actual cause of death, as opposed to the occurrence of death, problems of accuracy concerning reliability and validity appear. Secondly, comparisons on mortality are insensitive to differences among patients in the severity of the disease, and morbid episodes prior to death, including disability and handicap. Thirdly, mortality as a measure of outcome cannot apply to all situations, as disease causing death accounts for only a small proportion of total morbidity. Vuori's (1982 p. 88) comments in this regard are apposite: 'Mortality alone will hardly ever suffice to ascertain the impact or quality of health services. It may suggest that differences exist that are worthy of a closer look, but it is too crude a measure to provide guidelines

Figure 2.2: The Spectrum of Disease

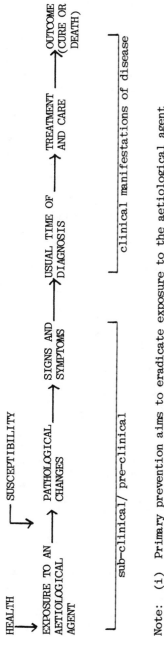

Note: (i) Primary prevention aims to eradicate exposure to the aetiological agent
      (ii) Secondary prevention (through screening and case-finding) aims at bringing forward the the usual time of diagnosis: that is, earlier on in the 'signs and symptoms' stage

for detailed priority setting and planning - let alone for assessing the quality of care given by a provider and for developing measures to improve his performance.' [4] In this light it is perhaps surprising that effectiveness studies have for so long addressed mortality as a key outcome variable. Obvious possibilities for extending attention beyond mortality exist (Figure 2.3), embracing particularly the issues of avoidable death and the quality of survival.

Rutstein et al (1974, 1976, 1980) present a straightforward, but valuable extension to such a simplistic mortality focus in evaluating health care, which has latterly attracted attention in the United Kingdom. (Charlton et al 1983) Their concern lies with the evaluation of the quality of care, in particular its effectiveness, in a general manner and also by disease categories. They argue that the basic stumbling block to quality assurance has so far been the lack of a measuring instrument, and it is to this end that their paper is addressed. If the objective of medical care is the maintenance of health and the prevention and treatment of disease, what is the value, asks Rutstein, of the increasing number of preventive and therapeutic agents, the many complex surgical procedures, the recommended changes in personal behaviour (for example, over diet and smoking) and the changing responsibilities and roles of health personnel? All would appear to need to be evaluated for their effectiveness and impact prior to their general use, something that has in general not occurred. (Cochrane 1972; McKeown 1976; Illsley 1980) But how is quality in terms of better health and the anticipated outcome of medical care to be measured?

Their argument is that the outcome of care (better health) can be defined in terms of the occurrence of unnecessary disease, disability or untimely death. (compare McKeown 1976 and Lalonde 1974) Such outcomes are termed 'sentinel' health events - warning signals. On their occurrence, their causes must be sought out. A sentinel event is then one that if everything had gone well in medical care the event would have been prevented or managed. The sentinel events themselves are established for each disease category after extensive discussion with clinical colleagues. A search must also be undertaken for who is responsible for the occurrence of the sentinel event. For example, is a case of diphtheria, rubella or poliomyelitis the responsibility of the

Figure 2.3: Simple Extensions to Mortality as a Measure of Outcome

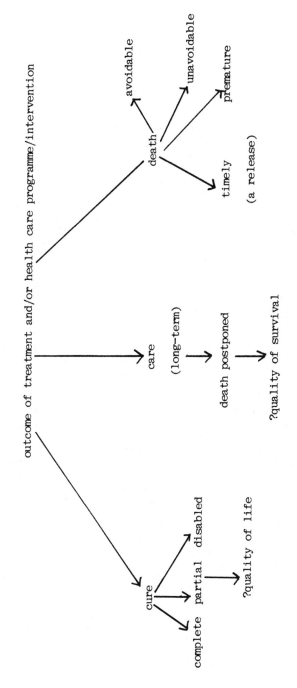

health authority for the lack of funding, or the health officials for not implementing the immunisation programme, or local opposition to clinics, or the family for not allowing the vaccination? Or again, is a death from lung cancer due to the patient's unwillingness or inability to give up smoking or to the government's policy on advertising and poisons, or to the absence of health education, and so on?

Rutstein's argument is then that the outcome of health care can be assessed by the identification and measurement of sentinel health events. Furthermore he argues that the health practitioner, the health authority, and/or the policy makers in government may have responsibility for the occurrence of sentinel events. The physician is at least partly responsible and so should seek to reduce their occurrence. It is of interest to note here that Rutstein's view of responsibility is at odds with that put forward by Weed (1973), who argues that the health provider is not responsible for the health outcome. Health outcomes are the preconditions of the health system; the question for the practitioner is only one of how well he has applied the rules. This ties in closely with Donabedian's (1980) notion of 'normative' validity, where the health practitioner is responsible not for the efficacy of the procedure used, but for selecting from those available according to the best professional opinion available.

Charlton et al (1983 p. 695) make use of Rutstein's approach when they select for study a small number of causes of untimely death, to analyse the variation in mortality among health authorities in England and Wales. The reversion to mortality as the outcome focus should be noted, '... the best routinely collected data in terms of availablity, economy, and completeness.' Their aim is apparently not to carry out a definitive evaluation but to see if any problems exist and thus to stimulate further enquiry as to cause. They find considerable variations in mortality, which remain after control for several social indicators (car ownership, housing and social class). Variation could of course still be explained by differences in the incidence of the illnesses, in the level of health provision, and in fact on all the potential causes of the illnesses, environmental, lifestyle, and genetic. This latter factor of the causation of illness and the limits on the impact of health services is discussed further in the next section of this Chapter.

While Rutstein and Charlton succeed in moving discussion a step further and partially away from the simplistic viewpoint of mortality, a more radical movement would seem to be called for, resulting in a measure of health that covers the morbidity resulting from an illness and in some instances mortality itself: indeed, a measure of health status regardless of illness. As the discussion concerning the definition of health concluded, a multi-dimensional measure is likely to be required, in order to embrace both the medical and the layperson's perceptions of health. In this light, objectives of health care programmes would need to be stated not only in terms of a reduction in the illness or an increase in the utilisation rate or the screening uptake, but also in terms of their implications for the functional and social levels of health of the individual (for example, in terms of the ability to carry out activities of daily living). The difficulties arise not in stating the objectives for the health programme in this way, but in generating valid and reliable measures. Any measure of health status will have to meet a range of issues which have been neatly summarised by Vuori:

> 'What constitutes a health problem? Who defines it? How can different problems be weighed? What are the objectives of the treatment of a given problem? Whose objectives have the highest priority? How can the priorities be quantified? How can problems that occur at different ages be handled? How can consequences that occur at different times be handled? What consequences of a given problem should be included? How can the different consequences be weighed?.' (Vuori 1982 p. 867)

The number of issues involved, plus the problems of data collection and availability,perhaps explains the lack of movement towards the actual use of any such indices.

The Ghana Health Assessment Team (1981) provides a halfway house solution. They adopted as a measure of health 'the number of healthy days of life which are lost through illness, disability and death as a consequence of disease'. To generate such a measure, data on the incidence of the illness, the case fatality rate and the extent and duration of disability are required. Their interest lay in examining the effect and impact of various health planning options and for arriving at resource allocation decisions. This approach has been widely discussed in the literature and used in connection with identifying the potential number of years of life lost through the occurrence of premature death from heart disease and cancer. (Romeder and McWinnie 1977; Tsai et al 1978, 1982) Culvez and Blanchet (1983) provide an illustration relating to Canada, devising a weighted index for different diseases and impairment states free of disability.

One attempt to develop a health status index is provided by Fanshel. (1972 p. 320) He defines health in relation to a functional conception of illness. 'A person is well if he is able to carry on his usual daily activities. To the extent that he cannot, he is in a state of dysfunction, or deviation from well-being.' From such an operational definition, Fanshel develops a continuum of 'states' of social dysfunction, ranging from 'well-being' in the World Health Organisation sense, 'discomfort' (symptoms but no significant reduction in ability to carry out one's daily activites), to 'confined, bedridden', and 'death' (absolute dysfunction). In all, eleven states are identified and an operational definition given to each. The aim is to classify individuals by their functional state and not by disease.

Having formulated a continuum measure of health, Fanshel goes on to develop a 'health status index' (HSI). His overall concern is not with the individual (a measure of individual healthiness) but with the population (an epidemiological concern). Accordingly, he assigns each state on the continuum a 'relative value' according to the individual and society as a whole. The values are then used as weights and applied to each state of dysfunction, leading to the HSI. The index is to be used for describing the health of the community in general terms, or for comparing the social effects of disease, or as a social indicator for reporting the health status of a population. It can also be used as a measure of output of the health services. So, Fanshel argues that if one accepts the aim of health services to be to improve the health status of the population, then the output of a health programme can be defined as '... the change in the functional history of the target population resulting from the intervention of the health programme (or health system).' (1972 p. 327)

Rosser and Watts (1972, 1978) and Rosser (1982) also proposed something similar but their attention lay on the measurement of hospital output, using two axes of disability and distress. Both of these are assessed by the health practitioner at the time of entry to the programme and at discharge. The general approach is one of comparing the health of the individual in terms of a stream of morbidity states resulting from the illness, from its onset until either recovery or death, which would occur in the absence of any medical care (or the actual programme under investigation) with the stream of morbidity states resulting from the actual treatment or health programme. The objective is that the point of recovery should occur earlier under the health programme than without it. A measure of its effect is then given by the difference in the (quantified) morbidity states, and a measure of its utility by a comparison of the utilities resulting under each stream.

Three points can be made on these two attempts to develop an index of health status. Firstly, at least in Fanshel's measure the individual's perception of health is given significance, in a joint position with that of the physician. Secondly, Fanshel points explicitly to the role of values in any definition of health. Interpreting if a person is on average worse off in moving from the well-being end of the continuum to the other, and weightings for the HSI are all value-based decisions. In terms of health services resources, one view would be to allocate resources in such a way as to move someone from an ill-healthy state, such as comatose or bedridden, to a healthy state, such as 'socially dissatisfied' or well-being itself. Thirdly, the approaches, while aimed like the Ghana Health Assessment Team at resource allocation and health services evaluation, also have relevance for assessing individual healthiness, and its changes over time. But as Fanshel observes, it is a moot point whether one measure of health is required. Rather, the chosen measure should depend on the actual purposes in hand, provided a breadth of perspective is adopted.

Several other examples of measures of community and individual health can be found in the liturature. For example, there is the Nottingham health profile. (Hunt et al 1980 and 1984) Here there is an explicit concern to take the layperson's own perception of health into account. It seeks to measure six areas: physical mobility, emotional reactions, pain, energy, sleep and social isolation. As a measure for assessing the effectiveness of a health programme it would appear to be potentially useful in evaluating impact from the consumer's point of view. It thus provides one way of taking the patient's perception into account in defining health need and health outcomes from a health intervention.

A more radical stance is advocated by Antonovksy (1980) in the development of his measure of health, the 'breakdown' concept. He argues that the dominant ideology of the pathogenic model, held by modern medical science and technology, with its response to a particular disease or clinical entity, must be challenged. The need is to orient research towards salutogenesis, that is, the origin and development of health. A health-disease continuum must be drawn up to identify where people lie, in the past, present and future, and to explore ways of moving them to the 'healthy' end of the continuum. Attention must therefore shift away from specific diseases and their risk indicators, towards trying to understand why and how some people manage to go through life with little suffering and pain, while others do not. His resultant measure of health status, the 'breakdown' concept comprises four dimensions. Firstly, there is a 'pain' dimension, a subjective phenomenon and so information on it must be gleaned from the individual. Variations in individuals' pain tolerance across cultures and over time can be anticipated. The exact cause of the pain may be emotional (the loss of a friend or a job) or due to an organic, physiological disorder. The second component is that of 'functional limitation', the capacity to undertake one's normal role or activities of daily living. Again, it is subjectively and individually defined. The third dimension concerns the 'prognostic implication' of the episode. At this point, questioning turns to the health practitioners, focussing on signs and symptoms, and associated prognosis. Three axes are addressed: the severity of the condition, its duration, and its social consequences. The final facet is the 'action implication' of ill-health. The physician is questioned concerning whether or not the condition requires health-related action, and if so what form.

Antonovsky's continuum measure of health builds on the earlier work of Fanshel (1972) and others such as Breslow (1972) and Cochrane (1972). It focusses on both the physician's and the individual's own viewpoint. Exactly why only the physician's comments on the social consequences of the illness are sought is unclear; for certainly the individual's own views would seem relevant too. But the monopoly of the health practitioner in defining health is questioned. It also addresses all three of Susser's dimensions of health. The resultant measure of health is dynamic, enabling observation of the movements of an individual or group over time. Finally, the measure would seem to generate reliable and valid data, and is not overly complex to use in practice. (Antonovsky 1973) [5]

Many options can then be seen to exist in relation to measuring health need and health status, the essential constitutent of a review of the effectiveness of a health programme or intervention. It has been argued that consideration must move from employing solely mortality; rather, a measure must take into account not only the health practitioner's viewpoint, but also that of potential consumers. This conclusion relates as much to measures of need and health status as to the process of effectiveness itself. The consumer's opinion and attitudes remain to be addressed and included.

DETERMINANTS OF ILLNESS AND THE ROLE OF HEALTH SERVICES

One fundamental problem in assessing the effectiveness of a health care programme is that of knowing whether the programme itself led to the improvement in the health status of the target population, or avoided a deterioration, or whether this was partially affected by some other factor in the population's environment or in general lifestyle, or to a spontaneous recovery. The question raised is that of attributable and relative effectiveness. It is instructive in this connection to consider the range of factors which can cause ill-health, and in this way to identify the potential (alternative) causal factors for any improvements in health noted after a health interventive programme. It also underlines the difficulty in this area because of the multifactoral nature of illness causation and, by implication, health itself, and the relative role of health services.

One useful model identifying possible causes

Figure 2.4:   The Diamond Model of Illness Causation

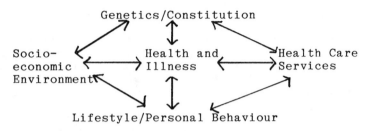

Note: The   arrows   indicate   inter-relationships   and
inter-actions.   In   particular   applications,   only
specific relationships/linkages will be observed.

of   illness   is depicted in Figure 2.4, where health
and illness are seen as determined by the effects of
four   sets of variables, in some form of interactive
and/or   independent   manner depending on the illness
under   consideration: the   host's   constitution;
personal   behaviour or lifestyle; the socio-economic
environment; and health and health related services.
All   of these factors can increase or ameliorate the
occurrence   of   illness,   and health itself.   Such a
model   has   been   put   forward explicitly by Lalonde
(1974)   in   his   concept   of   the   health field, and
implicitly   by   McKeown   (1976), Holland (1983), and
Long (1984).
       It   is worth looking at the components of these
sets   of   variables   in more detail.   Firstly, under
the   genetics/constitution factor are variables such
as   a   person's   age,   gender,   genetic   make-up and
immunological status, current nutritional state (and
the   effect   of   past   states),   and   constitutional
abilities   (both   predetermined   at   conception and
developed   during   life),   for   example to cope with
tension. (Antonovsky 1980)   Secondly,   the   health
care dimension points to the role of health services
provision   as   a   contributory factor to the delay in
the   development   and   prognosis   of an illness, and
sometimes   as   a   determinant itself, in the case of
iatrogenic   (doctor/health service induced) illness.
(Illich 1976)   In   other   words, this aspect covers
the   curative,   palliative   and   preventive roles of
health services, and includes factors such as health
education,   health   promotion,   screening,   and the
factor of access to, and equity of, health services.
Thirdly,   the   lifestyle or personal behaviour factor

34

points to the key role individual actions and
behaviour play on health. It embraces such
variables as smoking, diet, alcohol intake, and
other areas of personal choice. It also includes an
awareness of health services that are available and
perceptions of their value, and a person's own
perception of health and tolerance of pain. Aspects
of choice in a person's standard and way of living
are thus the focus. This may also involve reference
to other groups' behaviour, groups whom the
individual aspires to be like or become a member of.
Finally there is the aspect of the environment,
containing features of the socio-economic structure
of society. The factors of place of residence, air
pollution, occupation, exposure to occupational
hazards, social background and upbringing,
education, income and unemployment - as well as the
general structure of society - are all contained
under this heading. They can be distinguished from
the lifestyle dimension in that they are factors
over which the individual has in general little
control. The scope for personal choice is severely
restricted. The exact classification of a variable
as being under one dimension or another is of little
concern, compared to the need to note the
multifactoral nature of illness causation. Indeed,
to classify occupation as 'socio-economic
environment' or smoking as 'lifestyle' may be
politically contentious.

The underlying rationale of this model is that
not only is health and illness caused by an agent's
presence in a supportive environment and that the
host's susceptibility depends on resistance against
the agent, but that people's own actions and
behaviour in the broader socio-economic enviroment
affect their health. In addition, the provision and
access to health care can both positively (through
prevention, care and cure) and negatively (through
difficulty in access, or iatrogenic illness)
influence an individual's health state, as well as
in the very definition and perspective adopted on
the need or appropriateness of health provision.

One additional factor to the four identified in
the diamond model, perhaps contained under the
socio-economic enviroment is that of the political
and ideological dimension of the society. Knowledge
of the causes of ill-health may in some instances be
ignored or preventive action slow to emerge, due to
such factors as over-riding economic interests
(general industrial air pollution or exposure to
hazardous agents in the workplace), the effects on

employment and tax revenue (the example of tobacco and alcohol), and freedom of choice of individuals within the society (the example of flouridation). [6] Turning to the role of health services, this 'diamond' model of illness causation points to the fact that they are just one factor affecting the individual's or target population's state of health. They make a positive contribution to health status through the provision of effective health services, such as sound advice on health promotion, good quality hospital care, and so on. In contrast, they may contribute negatively in producing ill-health, through, for example, poor health education, inadequate and inappropriate health facilities, inequitable distribution of health services, and ineffective and iatrogenic health care in general. So in assessing the potential and actual effectiveness and impact of a health care programme it is therefore essential to consider the range of factors that may be contributing to the occurrence of the illness under review and thus to examine the appropriateness of the intervention or health care package.

It must be emphasised that in many instances the health care services are responding to the symptoms presented by patients and are not in themselves able to intervene to prevent exposure to the actual causes of the illness: for example, occupational illness following exposure to dangerous agents such as asbestos, coal dust or radiation; or exposure to lead following living near to a major traffic route; or depression among housewives; or heart disease where a critical role is played by the lifestyle factors of smoking and diet. The means of prevention do not always lie in the hands of the health service, but may be rather in the wider political environment, and in particular in the economic and political ideology dominant within society. (Navarro 1976; Doyal 1980) In this regard the role of health programmes and the issue of their effectiveness becomes of lessening significance, compared with consideration of how illness is caused by the general environment over which individuals have little or no control. (Vuori 1982)

In the context of assessing the effectiveness of a health service intervention or treatment regime, it is thus necessary to ask two questions. Firstly, what are the potential causes of the illness at which the programme is aimed; and secondly, what contribution can the health programme make to increasing the health of the target population? The model of illness causation is valuable in this regard only insofar as it elucidates the range of factors involved in affecting health besides health services. The basic point to note is that greater understanding of the causes of ill-health, irrespective of specific illnesses, is required in order to be able to intervene and prevent ill-health and also to satisfactorily treat more than just the resultant symptoms. It is important too to know how the various causes jointly determine ill-health. For example, do a bad diet and heavy smoking interact or merely bring about an additive increase in risk?

ISSUES OF DATA

In order to assess the effectiveness of a health care programme, it is essential for any measures of need or outcome, such as the various indices of health status discussed above, to provide data of sufficient quality and sensitivity that the actual effect of the service can be observed. Many commentators have drawn up checklists of criteria for quality assessment and assurance data to meet. (Donabedian 1980; Vuori 1982; Holland 1983) Most often mentioned are the features of validity (does it measure what it is meant to?) and reliability (is it consistent or repeatable over time and between observers?) of measurement, timeliness and the ready availability of the data, and the sensitivity (all those with the illness are diagnosed as ill) and specificity (all those without the illness are diagnosed as healthy) of the measures. Their importance is immediately apparent and only a few general comments are made here. In addition, attention will be drawn to Donabedian's concepts of causal and attributional validity.
Considerable play is made of the need for an indicator (of process or outcome) to be 'readily available' or 'easy to collect'. This factor would seem to go a long way to explaining the tendency to use mortality as a measure of outcome. However, the weight given to this criterion would seem to be excessive, and more strongly a gross misunderstanding of the principles and process of measurement. For a choice of indicator must depend on the extent to which it measures the concept or objective under consideration: the health state of the consumer prior to use of the programme or its alternative and the final state or outcome at the

completion of the programme. The reliability, validity, sensitivity and specificity of the indicator have a greater priority than that of ease of measurement or quantification and availability. Otherwise only spurious evaluations of effectiveness will take place.

The specificity of a measure of outcome is often problematic due to the fact that health care services are only one influence on health and only one influence on the individual's response to the services available. As Donabedian (1980 p. 107) points out, if an outcome can be attributed to prior health care there will still be difficulty in establishing which element of the process of care contributed to the failure to achieve the expected outcome, a point of considerable importance if performance is to be improved. As for sensitivity, two issues are of fundamental importance: firstly, how often a change in outcome is observed, and secondly the size of the change. For if the change in the outcome measure is likely to be small then it may be missed in measurement or explained away as due to problems of reliability and validity. Similarly if it is infrequent it may be missed unless a large number are observed. These problems are particularly likely to occur when using mortality as a measure of outcome. For as pointed out above, its sensitivity is moot.

Further to these comments on the validity of data is a fundamental principle of research validity, namely the basis for asserting that a process of care leads to a particular outcome. This is what Donabedian (1980 p. 102-6) describes as the issue of causal validity. [7] In the context of an outcome evaluation of the quality of care this refers to the causal linkage of a health programme (process of care) to a health outcome. To the extent that doubts exist over this linkage then problems arise over assessing the effectiveness of the programme, and more generally in using outcomes as indicators of the quality of care (similarly, for the use of processes as indicators of the quality of care). Taking this argument a stage further, knowledge of a valid causal link means only that it is possible to achieve a particular outcome under certain conditions. It thus does not mean that in a given situation the observed outcome has actually been produced by the antecedent process: for example, a patient's health improving spontaneously, or a baby dying unexpectedly. Many factors affect health in an individual, as indicated in the diamond

model outlined above. In this way, Donabedian
argues that as a first step it is essential to
establish that the particular outcome can be
attributed to the particular health programme. This
is what he calls the problem of attribution (the
issue of attributional validity, or external
validity/generalisation). So, once causal validity
has been established (X leads to Y under specific
conditions), then one must move on to see if it is
possible to argue for attributional validity (X
leads to Y in any situation). It is clear that many
rival causal factors may intervene to affect this
attribution process.

A final issue to mention in the context of
valid interpretations of data, is what Donabedian
(1980) describes as the issue of 'paradoxical
effects'. This refers to the difficulty of
explaining how it is possible for a population with
a generally poor state of health to be in receipt of
a good quality health service. He makes two points.
Firstly, this could be due to a 'survival effect'.
The higher the quality of health care services, the
more mortality will be postponed, the longer people
will survive, the greater the prevalence of
disability and the larger the number of chronically
ill people. Secondly, it could be explained by a
'discovery effect'. That is, where medical care is
of good quality the more disease and disability are
uncovered.

These comments regarding the general validity
of data and the need to be able to draw causal
conclusions regarding the link between a health
outcome and the health programme itself draw
attention to the need for good quality data sources,
and in many instances to the need to carry out a
specific research study in order to clarify and to
assess the effectiveness of the programme. Medical
records are unlikely to provide a comprehensive
picture of the care provided nor to contain data
that may be essential to an effectiveness review.
Participant observation studies (gathering the
relevant data as it happens) are one means of
obtaining relevant material. Indeed, it is more
than likely necessary to search widely for relevant
data. For example, Gray (1983) identifies a four box
model of health care: the hospital, the community,
informal care, and self-care. The further one moves
from the central box of hospital health services
provision the less data are available, and yet the
more relevant and appropriate such data are likely
to be in assessing need and exploring effective

interventions. Furthermore, rarely are data on health outcomes, even in the form of indications of prognosis, routinely recorded in medical records or extracted as management (monitoring) information. Even in the context of a major review of management information undertaken in the British NHS (the Körner (1982) reports), with its emphasis on minimum data sets (MDS), computerisation and ready access, no data were recommended for inclusion and collection on health outcome following a health intervention or process of care, health status of the community, or health status prior to any health intervention or treatment regime. As important an issue, though, is that of knowing precisely what it is that one is trying to assess and measure, and to design a study in such a way that causal conclusions can be drawn.

ASSESSING EFFECTIVENESS: SOME METHODOLOGICAL ISSUES

Effectiveness studies focus on the outcome of a health care programme. A clear definition of its objective is required. The question normally posed is whether the intervention (the health care programme) can alter the outcome of the natural history of the disease at which it is aimed. (Holland 1983) Major problems faced in assessing effectiveness are those of the measurement of the outcome state, prior to the programme and after it, and then attributing the change in outcome status to the programme itself. Discussion now turns to explore some of the methodological principles to be followed in attempting to assess effectiveness, and to examine some possible approaches to such assessment. It is not the intention to cover the various research designs in any detail, as these are already well described in the literature. (Campbell 1969; Cook and Campbell 1979; Holland 1983) The health outcome of a programme, following Rosser and Watts (1972), can be defined as the difference between a patient's health status following (and during, as appropriate) an episode of health care in comparison with an estimate of the patient's health status in the absence of such a programme. The difference between the observed state (treatment-induced, at least hypothetically) and the expected state (in the absence of treatment) may of course vary both during the illness, and afterwards. That is, outcome itself is a function of time; in the long term, the greater the time since the treatment or intervention, the less difference is likely to be observed in the two states. The outcome state can be further refined to differentiate between the absolute outcome at a given time (the simple difference between the two states), relative outcome (the ratio of the two), and comparative outcome (the two states compared relate to two different types of health programme – that is, a focus on relative effectiveness) (Association of Medical Records Officers 1983).

What then are the minimum requirements, methodologically speaking, in order to assess the effectiveness of a health care programme? The simplest design which is likely to be of any value can be described as follows:

$$O_1 \qquad T \qquad O_1$$

$$O_2 \qquad \qquad O_2$$

where T stands for the exposure to the treatment or programme; O_1 stands for the observation of one group, and O_2 for observation of a second group. In other words, two groups of patients or consumers are studied, one of whom participates in the health programme, the other does not. The health status (outcome state) is measured for both groups on a minimum of two occasions, at least prior to the treatment and after it.

Such a design will only be of value under a number of conditions. Firstly, the two groups must be comparable in every respect prior to exposure to the health care programme. Secondly, clear, unambiguous, reliable and valid measurements must be made of the outcome states. Thirdly, the difference between the two groups must be able to be inferred as being due solely to the different health care experience and to nothing else, such as the effect of alternative causes of changes in health status (for example, due to the operation of factors indicated in the diamond model of illness causation outlined above), or spontaneous improvements in health status due solely to the interest taken in the participants (the so called Hawthorne effect), and so on. In other words, the study must be designed and undertaken such that causal validity (in Donabedian's terms) is assured. [8]

These conditions are difficult to meet, but are nonetheless essential in order to be confident that the changes in health status observed can actually be said to be caused by the programme. In research design terms, the study must have high internal validity. Possible options in research methods are the following designs: a randomised controlled trial, a retrospective case-comparison study, a prospective case-comparison study (a cohort design), or an ethnographic study using observation in the natural setting where hypotheses of the health programme's effects are systematically assessed through the use of the comparative method, involving the search for confirming and denying instances and the minimising and maximising of differences between comparison groups. (Glaser and Strauss 1968; Cook and Reichardt 1979; Hammersley and Atkinson 1983; and Long 1984)

Each of these options has its advantages and limitations. In the randomised controlled trial, control over all other variables is obtained through the use of randomisation. In this way the two groups are made to be explicitly identical and comparable prior to exposure to the programme. No factor is allowed to vary except the treatment. Thus causal validity is assured. But this is only the theory. In practice, there are several difficulties. It is not always possible ethically to randomly allocate people to the two groups. The study is also rarely if ever conducted in an isolated laboratory setting; so, other factors outside of the control of the researcher can enter and affect the situation. The extended time-scale of an evaluation experiment also allows more opportunities for other variables to intervene. In any case, Hawthorne and other experimenter-induced effects can still operate to confound the research findings, leading on to the option of double blind procedures. The measurement of the outcome too may not be unequivocal. Although mortality is, it is likely to be inappropriate and insensitive. Finally, the longer term effects of the programme, and any side-effects, may not be observed because the observation time of the study was too short, the effects thus arising after the study was completed. Further, if the study period was longer, other factors might be suggested as causes of the outcome. [9]

In the other mentioned designs similar problems exist. For the retrospective case-comparison study, the comments on measurement apply with the added complication of recall bias, and the possible inadequacies of medical and other health records. There may also be difficulties in obtaining comparability in the case and comparison series (the cases are those who have participated in the health programme) with obvious consequential problems for causal validity. In the prospective case comparison design, the problem of ethics of randomisation disappears (though as in any effectiveness study the ethics of the study itself still remain). The major stumbling block again is that of assuring the equivalence of the two groups, and controlling for the effects of other variables that might affect the health outcome states. Finally, the problems faced in an ethnographic study (on lines similar to that of a prospective case-comparison study) relate to its expense in terms of time and manpower and doubts over the 'objectivity' of the resultant data. But in the context of 'softer' measurement with the development of the health status indices it may be a very valuable option to pursue. [10]

From these brief comments it is quite apparent that establishing a sound research design to study effectiveness is problematic. Pointing to threats to the validity of research is not an argument against evaluation. On the contrary, the evaluator needs to be aware of potential threats and thus to take steps to minimise (eradication may be impossible) their effect in a particular study. Indeed, evaluation is essential. For not only is it unethical on some occasions to randomise or to withhold a treatment one believes to be effective, even though it has not be demonstrated from research, it is also unethical to provide a treatment whose efficacy is dubious or non-existent. Such an argument can be extended to the more common situation where one does not know for sure what the effects of a particular programme are. Evaluation is thus paramount especially prior to the introduction of a new treatment (when it is in any case ethically and professionally easier) and also in the context of the many unproved current practices. (Cochrane 1972; Illsley 1980) It should of course be noted that a particular treatent may be self-evidently effective without the need for formal research on its effectiveness: for example, the use of penicillin for pneumococcal pneumonia. (Miettienen 1983)

One issue that must be addressed is whether it is necessary to carry out a formal research study to assess the effectiveness of a health programme or whether it is possible to evaluate it as a by-product of normal operational practice. The answer lies in the nature and value of the available data bases and the attention given within them to include data on outcome. Medical records are unlikely, unless special consideration has been given to the issue, to contain the necessary data on changes in morbidity and recovery states, or to contain measurement of the health status of patients prior to treatment. This point was noted above in relation to developments in data systems in the British NHS, following the implementation of the Körner Steering Committee recommendations. Death is the only certain factor to be recorded, an insensitive index in most cases. Further, depending on the length of time of the evaluation in relation to the duration of the patient's illness episode, medical records may simply not be a relevant source of information. For example, if evaluation is to occur for a hospital treatment and to continue for one month after discharge from the hospital, the records are unlikely to contain any data relating to the patient's time in the community except for any attendance at an outpatient clinic. The problems will occur in both a retrospective and prospective evaluation where medical records are the source of data. It is thus necessary in general to ensure that the medical records are expanded for the period of the evaluation study, or that special records are created for the studied patients. In this latter case a formal research study is in effect being undertaken.

Three points are worth noting here. Firstly, assessing effectiveness as part of a performance review system is not a one-off activity. Accordingly, regular monitoring systems are required, implying the need for continuous records of health outcomes, even after causal validity has been proved. Secondly, in the context of the British NHS, while the Körner information initiative does not require outcome data as part of the minimum data sets, there is nothing to stop health practitioners from collecting such data, adding them to the information system. Such an initiative can only be encouraged. Thirdly, and on a more sanguine note, there is doubt as to whether, even if relevant and accurate data on health outcome were routinely (or in an ad hoc manner) collected, the health practitioners and policy makers have the will and commitment to act upon the evidence. In other words, one can comment sceptically that rational decision making and planning is not the norm in health service decision making, professional or even self interests holding greater sway.

Two general principles to assist in formulating

a sound research design to study effectiveness can
be advanced. Firstly, valid and reliable
measurement are essential employing a meaningful
measure. For there is little to be gained from
employing an insensitive measure of outcome just
because of difficulties in generating a valuable
health status index. Secondly, in the context of
interventive research, the principle of information
efficiency (Miettinen 1981; Kleinbaum et al 1982;
and Long 1984) recommends the use of a 'high risk'
group as the study's focus. For it is in such a
group that the greatest effect of a health
intervention will be observed. Half of the group
will then receive the treatment, the other half
receiving the alternative (the standard treatment),
or a placebo. Thirdly, the study must generate
reseach findings that are causally valid. In
addition, one wants to be able to generalise from
such a setting to others, and thus to be able in
general to attribute the change in health status to
the health service intervention.
    One of the major difficulties of interventive
research arises from the very nature of health
services, that is, the imperative to focus a service
toward high risk consumers. As Miettinen (1983)
points out, the study of intended effects of health
care programmes and therapies is problematic on two
counts: the difficulty of identifying cause and
effect; and the problem of ruling out alternative
explanations of the data. Contained in these
problems is the issue of confounding: that is, a
variable that distorts or confounds the relation
between the treatment and the outcome. The very
logic of the study of intended effects is that there
is a need for intervention to bring about a desired
change in the health outcome. Without the
intervention, the expected health outcome is
undesirable; the worse the expected outcome, the
greater the desire for intervention. This leads to
a situation where the very fact of high risk or poor
prognosis constitutes an 'indication' for
intervention. 'Where such an indication guides the
use of intervention, it constitutes a confounder.'
(Miettienen 1983 p. 268) [11] The usual effect
Miettinen argues is in fact negative; that is, it
reduces the effect (the size of the relationship) of
the treatment on the outcome. Care must then be
exercised in evaluation research for such
indications and attempts made to control for their
influence.
    As a final comment on possible research designs

to assess the effectiveness of a health intervention, three general approaches are worthy of mention. Firstly, there are the techniques of economic appraisal of cost-benefit analysis, and cost effectiveness analysis. In the former, attention lies on quantifying the benefits (to the patients and the community) of the health care programme and comparing these to the costs of the programme. The basic problems to be faced are those relating to the measurement and quantification of the benefits and their restatement in monetary units to compare to the costs. In this context effectiveness is then viewed in terms of a favourable benefit to cost ratio.

A second approach is one put forward by Illsley (1980) and can be described as a holistic approach. He argues that it is particularly applicable to situations where the method of the controlled trial cannot apply, due to ethical difficulties over randomisation and problems over generating a single measurable index of outcome and where there are a multiplicity of actors involved all of whose perspectives ought to be taken into account. He presents two examples of research carried out in the way he is suggesting. Firstly in the context of adeno-tonsillectomy, pathways to decisions over whether to perform this operation, and decision choices and criteria employed, have to be spelt out. The emphasis lies on evaluating the whole process of care. Secondly, in the situation of antenatal care he argues for the need to look at the several components of care. In both, many actors are involved (patients, nurses, general practitioners, and hospital physicians), all with potentially differing perceptions, each requiring to be examined and compared. While Illsley's approach clearly addresses the process of care, its basic logic is applicable to outcome evaluation. For the complexity of the care process cannot be ignored.

The third approach is one commented on at length by Donabedian (1980) and put forward originally be Freeborn and Greenlick (1973). [12] Their argument is that in the assessment of performance the twin aspects of effectiveness and efficiency must be examined. Looking only at their comments on effectiveness, they divide these into two parts. Firstly, there is the need to assess 'technical' effectiveness. This involves a focus on the structure of the health system providing the care, the process of providing the care - divided into its accessibility, the performance of providers, and the continuity of care - and the technical outcome of care. Secondly, there is the aspect of 'psychosocial' effectiveness, which is divided into patient satisfaction and provider satisfaction. As Donabedian points out, this leads to the interesting possibility of distinguishing client-related or client-preferred and provider-related outcomes. In this way, they draw attention to the value of studying both attitudes and behaviours as a way of learning about the satisfaction of providers and consumers. It is interesting to note that this suggests the use of the ethnographic research style with its emphasis on exploring the formal and explicit and the hidden and the tacit versions of reality.

A CHECKLIST TO REVIEW EFFECTIVENESS

The discussion so far has pointed to the dilemmas faced in designing studies to explore the effectiveness of a health care programme or intervention. Problems of data, measurement, need and outcome, confidence in assuming causal validity, as well as the problem of attributional validity once the studied procedure comes into wider use: all such difficulties require resolution in any study. Perfect research designs and practice, or perfect continuous monitoring systems for quality assurance or performance review are not possible. However, understanding likely difficulties and threats to validity should not limit attempts to assess effectiveness. The argument has been that health status indices must be drawn up, to overcome the narrowness and insensitivity of mortality as an outcome measure. Such indices too must try to take account of the potentially varying perspectives of the consumers, health practitioners and policy makers.

In the final section of this Chapter, a matrix of questions building on the preceding discussion is drawn up to assist in the process of reviewing the effectiveness of a health programme or intervention. Table 2.2 lists some dimensions and topics which are important to explore in any review of a study on effectiveness. [13] The first three items indicated provide the context of the health programme or intervention under consideration. The importance of specifying the way the service is delivered relates to the ease of replicating the intervention in other settings and to the field of

Table 2.2: Evaluating Effectiveness Studies: Some Critical Questions

1. What is the area of the intervention? What are the illness categories or client groups?

2. What potential intervention/health programme is evaluated? What are its objectives?

3. How is the programme being delivered? What are the conditions under which the intervention is being assessed?

4. What is the target population? Differentiate the potential recipients (likely users) and those in greatest need who may not take up the programme.

5. What is the outcome measure? How is it defined and measured? What dimensions of health are addressed? Is the measurement valid and reliable?

6. What is the general research design? What type of study is it? Are confounding factors controlled? Is causal validity achieved? Is the study size sufficient?

7. What factors are probable causes of the phenomenon to which the intervention is directed? What role might they have in the study on any observed changes in health status?

8. Are there any wider effects on the programme in a social and political sense, either intended or unintended? Identify and explore their impact and relevance to the overall worth of the intervention.

9. What attention is given to the consumer's and the health practitioner's satisfaction with the service/programme? Identify their viewpoints.

10. What is the cost of the intervention (leading to a concern with efficiency and cost effectiveness)?

11. How can the intervention or mode of delivery be improved to increase its effectiveness? Or, what steps are necessary to curtail the programme if it is found to be ineffective?

generalisation. As for the elaboration of the
target population, it is valuable to differentiate
the potential recipients of a programme from those
who, on the basis of a clinical and/or social
definition, actually are in need of it. Ways of
ensuring that those in need receive and use the
service may then be more easily identified. In
relation to question five it is necessary to
identify the way the outcome is defined and measured
and to assess its reliability and validity.
Depending on how the programme's objective is
specified it may be valuable to look both at the
health and health related outcome: that is, effects
of the programme on the patient's wider social
involvement. Under this heading attention should
also be directed at the breadth of definition of the
health outcome and its consideration of the
varying perspectives of the key actors.
    The subsequent areas identified in the Table
relate to features of the study itself. Under the
heading of research design it is critical to assess
whether or not causal validity is present: that is,
are alternative causes and other confounding factors
controlled for and thus not operating in the
research setting. The issue of sample size is also
important in giving confidence over the
generalisability of the study and thus its relevance
for wider health practice (attributional validity),
and over the ability to differentiate rival
hypotheses (the notion of power in statistics).
Attention must then turn to the extent to which
the health services can affect the illness under
review, or improve the health of the target
population: that is, to spell out possible
alternative causes of the phenomenon in question and
thus to consider the role and potential impact of
these factors on any health status change observed.
It is also important to consider the wider effects
that the programme may have in other areas, in
particular any that may be unintended (for example,
an unwanted effect of a drug or operative procedure,
in encouraging the multiplication of cancer cells),
and to consider the views of the consumer (client
satisfaction). Once the effectiveness of a
procedure is assured, attention can turn to the area
of cost, linking to the concept of efficiency, the
topic of Chapter Three. The final question aims to
ensure that any review is constructive. In this
instance, the concern is that of how to improve the
effectiveness of the health programme, or if it is
ineffective, to identify what steps must be taken to

curtail the service and replace it with something more appropriate, and then to implement them.

Such a set of review questions can be applied quite easily to studies on the effectiveness of a health programme. For example in Mather's study (1976) of the place of treatment for patients who have suffered an acute myocardial infarction, the concern was to explore whether patients treated in their own homes would fare as well as those treated in a coronary care unit and general medical ward. The outcome measure employed is crude (mortality at 28 and 330 days) and only gives attention in effect to the organic dimension of health; the quality of survival is not addressed. As for the research design, a randomised controlled trial is employed leading to control over relevant confounding variables such as time until first receipt of medical care, and previous history of cardiovascular disease. However, the study is plagued with the problem of the self-fulfilling prophecy (Hawthorne effect) in relation to the type and quality of care provided by the participating GPs and hospital physicians, and the effect of other potentially confounding factors such as social class. Doubt must surround the causal validity of the study because of the effect of these uncontrolled variables, but only to the extent that they affect the treatment groups differentially. There is too some concern over the randomisation proportion; for not everyone who had had an acute myocardial infarction could be included in the study for ethical reasons. In terms of the wider effects of the intervention, it is addressed to the issue of the need (and cost implications) for a CCU; there is also the question of the expectations of the community regarding hospital care. The question of cost is not addressed in this paper, but the implication is that home care is likely to be cheaper. No attention is given to the issue of satisfaction either of the patients and relatives or of the providers. As for improvements to the study in order that the relative and cost effectiveness can be more completely assessed, attention must be given to control for the confounding factors mentioned, and to explore the cost dimension. [14]

This checklist of questions is specifically designed to evaluate available studies exploring the effectiveness of the use of manpower groups, patterns of health delivery, or potential interventive programmes. That is, it is directed at

Table 2.3: Key Questions for Reviewing the Effectiveness of a Service [15]

A. Long Term Objectives and Measures of Outcome
1. What are the objectives of the health programme, intervention, or manpower group being reviewed? Identify health and health related objectives.
2. How can their achievement be assessed. Draw up (quantitative) indicators and measures of health outcome.

B. Current Service and Need
1. What is the level, type and extent of the current service?
2. Who gets the service?
3. Who needs it?
4. What gaps exist? What limits (financial, manpower, technological) on it are there?

C. Comparison of the Ideal and the Actual
1. What is the impact of the current service on its stated objectives (A.1), in terms of the indicated measures of outcome (A.2)?
2. What evidence is there for changes in health status as being due to the health programme (the problems of causal, and attributional validity).

D. Areas for Modification and Implementation
1. How can the impacts of the programme be increased? Identify any wider social or political issues raised (such as professional views, or governmental policy).
2. Who will attempt to implement the recommended programme changes? How will this be done?

E. Cost
1. What is the cost of the current service, in absolute terms and in relation to changes in outcome?
2. What will the cost be if greater (specify its magnitude) impact is achieved?

Source: Freely adapted from Clayden, 1984

51

specially commissioned research studies on
effectiveness. Even without undertaking a major
research study, the effectiveness of current and
possible health provision can be assessed. Table
2.3 present a rearrangement of these questions to
this end. (Clayden 1984) It is split into five
parts: identification of the objectives of the
health programme and ways to assess their
achievement; a review of current service provision,
and the need for the service; a comparison of
current service provision, and the need for the
service; a comparison of the current service with
the stated objectives to assess its impact; ways to
improve the level of impact; and cost efficiency.

Such a checklist poses a challenge to health
providers, in terms of clearly specifying the
objectives of the service provided, identifying
potential indicators to assess their achievement,
and quantifying and justifying the level of impact
of current service provision. For example, in
reviewing services for the elderly, two objectives
identified by health providers using this checklist
of questions were 'to keep the elderly out of
hospital as long as possible', and 'to improve
community support for the elderly, and for the
carers of the elderly'. Translating such long term
aims into quantitative indicators was difficult; one
indicator argued for was 'the proportion of 65/75/85
year olds who were admitted to hospital for other
than medical conditions'. As for the impact of
current services on these objectives, the group
commented that 'in particular we rarely get this far
on (in our thinking and analysis)'. Another example
based on another group's work, relating to primary
health care is depicted in Table 2.4. As a final
comment, it is worth noting the article by Smith and
Haggard (1982), which discusses how a not dissimilar
approach was adopted in Cambridge Health Authority
in the British NHS.

CONCLUSION

The main concern of this Chapter has been to
demonstrate the need to explore the effectiveness of
health programmes and then to begin to undertake an
evaluation of health services, relating health needs
to desired health outcomes. It has been argued that
data on relevant and sensitive measures of health
outcome are required, with attention being given to
shift towards the development of reliable and valid

Table 2.4: Reviewing Primary Health Care ...

Objectives	Assessing Their Achievement	...	Who Gets Service?	Who Needs Service?	...	What is Level of Impact of Current Service?	Evidence? ...
A. DIRECT HEALTH							
1. To prevent ill health; to decrease preventable illness	Incidence (mortality and morbidity)		THOSE WHO PRESENT FOR TREATMENT SELF OVER	INVERSE CARE LAW / BLACKS / WORKING CLASS etc. / OLD / WHO REPORT		'Some'	Data difficult to obtain. A few surveys (eg Acheson, for London; or Wood, for Manchester)
2. To promote health	% knowing about (eg) healthy diet sales of food-stuffs etc					'Little'	
3. To increase validity and reliability of diagnosis							Need more information (so objective five); education of the profession too
4. To improve access to PHC; to identify pop-ulation in 'need'	Use for emergencies (in comparison with A/E department) waiting time, home visits (%)					'Little'	
...							
B. HEALTH RELATED							
5. To improve information base	Morbidity Review (including satis-faction surveys)					'Little'	
...							

Key: ... denotes parts missed out

53

indices of health status, taking into account the
varying perspectives of the relevant actors. Once
this is completed the next difficulty is that of
designing and undertaking a sound study to assess
the effectiveness of the programme. A comparison
group is essential, one that is similar in every
respect except the treatment regime. From the
health practitioner's viewpoint, such a study would
then have to be reviewed, prior to the utilisation
of its findings. The checklist of Table 2.2 is of
relevance here. However, the more general case will
be one where the actual service provided has not
been researched in any systematic manner, and thus
the health provider will need to set about
evaluating its effectiveness from first principles,
following a checklist such as Table 2.3.

The evaluation of health services must be
founded in the first instance on effectiveness.
Once effectiveness has been confirmed, attention
can turn to the efficiency of the services provided.
Plotting, these two aspects for potential health
programmes for a disease category, say, against one
another provides a useful means for identifying the
extent to which the target area of an effective and
efficient programme is achieved. Evaluation also
embraces the concept of acceptability, the subject
of Chapter Four. At present the most unaddressed
area is that of the consumer's viewpoint, in terms
of defining health needs, measures of health
outcome, the effectiveness of services, costs of
service, and satisfaction with them.

But reviewing and assessing effectiveness,
efficiency, and acceptability, however sound the
data and studies are, has to meet one final barrier
before it becomes part of clinical and health
practice: that is, the political dimension,
involving a willingness to address these issues, and
to implement the results of any research or
systematic evaluation. Issues such as professional
self-interest; a willingness to look beyond one's
own area of activity to the wider good of the
community; the possibility of shifting resources
from the highly technical, expensive, and perhaps
effective but costly glamour services to addressing
the more mundane needs of the wider community; and
willingness to consider influencing and acting upon
these factors outside of the health services field
of activity, which affect the health status of the
population it serves (for example, to influence
government policy on smoking, alcohol and food
subsidies) all involve an action implication and

political commitment. Without such an imperative, evaluation as an activity becomes a sterile exercise, being undertaken for its own sake, without any consequent improvement in the health status of the community.

NOTES

1. See for example, Antonovsky (1980); or Stacey (1977). For an extended discussion of issues surrounding the definition of, and perspectives on, health and illness, see Long (1984).
2. There is, for example, the British survey of Wadsworth (1971), or Antonovsky's (1980) review for the USA. See too the various reports since 1976 of the General Household Survey (OPCS 1983).
3. See also p. 71 where Holland presents a slightly different model, exploring medically defined need in relation to (individually) perceived need and actual use of health services.
4. See also Doll (1974).
5. For an extended discussion of possible measures of community health, see Long (1984).
6. See, for example, Alderson (1982); Bross (1982); Doll and Peto (1981); Doyal and Epstein (1983); Long (1984); Oldham and Newell (1977); and Townsend and Davidson (1982).
7. Donabedian's notion of causal validity is equivalent to that of 'internal validity' employed in texts on research methods.
8. That is, the study has internal validity. For discussion of potential problems in research design, and alternative approaches, see Long (1984).
9. This is often a source of bias in a cohort design, of which a randomised controlled trial is an example. See Miettinen (1981); and Long (1984).
10. For a discussion of ethnography, see Hammersley and Atkinson (1983); McCall and Simons (1969); or Long (1984).
11. In a study of unintended effects, one can randomise. This is only possible in a study of intended effects if a randomised controlled trial design is ethically feasible. For a discussion of some relevant issues on ethics, see Hiller (1981) and Long (1984).
12. Donabedian (1980 pp. 93-97) provides his own extension of Freeborn and Greenlick's framework.
13. Broader checklists for assessing the general validity of research are available. See

Stern (1979); Sapsford and Evans (1979); or Long (1984.

14. For a further discussion of Mather's study see Long (1984).

15. To complete such a review of a service, additional questions relating to efficiency (Chapter 3) acceptability (Chapter 4) and aspects of organisational behaviour (Chapter 5) need to be added.

Chapter 3

EFFICIENCY IN HEALTH CARE

Ray Brooks

Efficiency has been likened to a state of grace:
something to which all aspire, but which few achieve
and then only fleetingly. Certainly, efficiency
seems to be universally regarded as a good thing,
but what is it? The purpose of this Chapter is to
give a brief description of four different economic
concepts of efficiency, allocative, distributive,
dynamic, and managerial, and to consider how each of
these relates to the field of health care, including
some of the difficulties involved in their
application. In addition, the various financial
methodologies and their relationship to the
different economic concepts of efficiency are
discussed. The Chapter ends with a comparison of
the economist's viewpoint on the concept of
efficiency with that of the accountant, together
with a summary of the main differences between
the four types of efficiency.

ALLOCATIVE EFFICIENCY

The notion of allocative efficiency is derived from
the nineteenth century work of Pareto (1972), whose
'principle of optimality' holds that there is a
point at which the pattern of consumption of goods
and services in a society cannot be rearranged to
make one individual better off without making
another worse off. In classical economic theory,
just such an arrangement of consumption will be
produced by the functioning of perfect competition
in a free market (see for instance Friedman 1980).
The conditions for such competition are held to
include many small firms, the absence of collusion
between suppliers, the equivalence of products
offered as between suppliers, the self-interest of

all actors in the market, the mobility of consumers, a level of knowledge on the part of the consumers such that additional knowledge could not improve their decisions, free entry to and exit from the market, free movement of market prices, and the absence of external influence on the conditions of exchange.

It is evident that the existence of such conditions is the exception rather than the rule. To use examples from the health care field, it is clear that professional licensure laws prevent free entry to the medical market, that consumers are relatively immobile and unable to seek preferred health care services, and that consumer knowledge of the content and effectiveness of such services is largely absent. It is these real world imperfections which have led analysts such as Galbraith (1963) to suggest that producer, rather than consumer, sovereignty is the prevalent condition.

Perhaps the most important technique which responds to these points is cost-benefit analysis, defined as a way of

> assessing the desirability of projects where it is important to take a long view (in the sense of looking at repercussions in the further, as well as the near, future) and a wide view (in the sense of allowing side effects of many kinds on many persons ... etc.); i.e. it implies the enumeration and evaluation of all the relevant costs and benefits. (Prest and Turvey 1965)

The steps involved in cost-benefit analysis are summarised in Table 3.1. Logically, cost benefit analysis implies an infinite number of comparisons of the subject of the study with every alternative way of spending the resources, and is part of the intellectual foundation of the concept of zero-based budgetting. Clearly, this is not practicable, and most cost-benefit studies in health care have concentrated on determining a benefit - cost index for one treatment (see for instance Hagard et al 1976), or on comparing the indices for a small number of alternative treatments for a particular disease (see for instance Weisbrod 1982). In the health care field, the link with effectiveness is an obvious one. 'Alternative' may encompass such questions as the timing and location of treatment, as well as its

Table 3.1: Steps in Cost-Benefit Analysis

1. Lay out the alternative programmes for evaluation.

2. Specify the resource requirements of each programme.

3. Count all of the economic costs and benefits of each programme. Those costs will include both the cash costs and the opportunity costs involved in the use of a resource, whilst excluding sunk costs. The benefits will include all of those devolving to the community, as well as upon the patient.

4. Discount the costs and benefits at the relevant cost of capital (this may be the social rate of discount, see Drummond 1980).

5. Compare the discount totals and identify all alternatives which demonstrate a positive value of benefits over costs.

content.
Even this more restricted approach offers considerable methodological difficulties. Firstly, all costs and benefits are to be taken into account; the longer the period and the more diverse the actors upon whom these fall, the greater the difficulty. Nevertheless, it is the essence of cost-benefit analysis that an attempt is made to take account of all socially relevant outcomes including those 'externalities' which fall upon those other than the intended beneficiaries or payers (such as patients' relatives). Secondly, costs should reflect opportunity cost: what opportunities are foregone as a result of a particular decision? Thirdly, the calculation of costs require the estimation (in the health field) of a value for such intangibles as pain and suffering, as well as a decision about appropriate discount rates to reflect different timings of costs and benefits. Fourthly, benefits may also be largely incommensurable. Fifthly, the focus should be upon benefits obtained and costs incurred in one increment or decrement of the level of service provided. (See Mooney 1983 for an example of the application of marginal analysis to residenial accommodation for the elderly.) Finally, health service statistics and accounts are

often not kept in a form which allows their use in this kind of analysis; they may for instance be incident rather than patient-related. (Hagard et al 1976 p. 50) This is not to say that no progress has been made. Sometimes it will be enough merely to indicate the existence of a cost or benefit. (Weisbrod 1982 pp. 809-10) Data can be improved in some respects; for instance, in Britain the Körner Report (Steering Group on Health Service Information 1982) will lead to the provision of additional patient-centred data, though of course such arrangements cannot capture indirect benefits.

Cost-benefit analysis is therefore of considerable potential value in the health care field, and has been used to examine such issues as the best mix of kidney transplantation and home and hospital dialysis (Buxton and West 1975), surgical versus scleropathy treatment for varicose veins (Piachaud and Weddell 1972), screening for neural tube defects (Hagard et al 1976), and outpatient versus inpatient treatment for the mentally ill. (Weisbrod 1982)

The value of cost-benefit analysis in an application to improve allocative efficiency is that it can give a local optimisation within the limits of the studied areas, ceteris paribus. Such a localised study offers the advantage of concentration on particular areas of concern, as has been seen. However, the technique must be seen in the light of the 'theory of second best', which holds that the absence of any one of the primary requirements for perfect competition means that it is neither necessary nor desirable to satisfy the remaining requirements, and that it cannot be assumed that policies aimed at reducing market imperfections will necessarily increase overall welfare. The theory has been mathematically demonstrated by Henderson and Quandt (1971 pp. 286-288). Thus even if a localised cost-benefit study can overcome the problem of externalities it must still pay due attention to the 'second best' problems.

In summary, the concept of allocative efficiency may be applied to health care at two distinct levels. The first level raises the question of whether the resources devoted to health care within a society would produce greater benefits if allocated to some other sector of the economy, and of course vice versa. This requires a major study of both the supply side and the demand side of all economic sectors, a not insubstantial piece of work! In effect, the study of allocative efficiency at this level is everything, or it is nothing.

The second level concerns the allocation of new resources within the health care system. The 'theory of second best' indicates that reducing just some allocative imperfections will not necessarily increase total welfare. Nevertheless, a number of economists in the United States have held that it is desirable to reduce market imperfections in order (inter alia) to improve allocative efficiency (see for example Enthoven 1978).

DISTRIBUTIVE EFFICIENCY

The theory of distribution considers the virtue of an organisation's arrangements for the distribution of its goods and services. The efficiency of these arrangements for distribution depends upon the structure of the organisation, its channels for distribution and upon the access afforded to consumers by health care facilities. There have broadly been two approaches by economists to the study of distributive efficiency. The first approach has been to compare and contrast the organisational (structural) arrangements on the supply side of the market. The second approach recognises the need to judge the 'equity' or 'justice' of those arrangements and attempts to include relevant factors in its analysis.

Structural analysis has been well developed since Joan Robinson's (1933 p. 4) pioneering work, which recognised that 'the real world (did) not fulfill the assumptions of perfect competition'. This approach led to the development of the concepts of monopoly, duopoly, monopsony, and market power. All are main issues of concern to those public bodies that regulate markets in general, and the market for health care in particular.

The 1974 Reorganisation of the British NHS is a clear example of government-imposed change in organisational structure which was expected to produce improvements in efficiency. This approach depended upon the government's direct control of organisation arrangements. The U.S. approach differs, in that control is exercised via anti-trust legislation, regulation, certification, tax incentives/disincentives and not least by reimbursement systems. The actual form of organisation is not controlled.

In his recent analysis of the US health care

system Starr (1982 pp. 429 ff) noted five separate dimensions of economic and organisational analysis. His first dimension was the not-for-profit/for-profit range of legal structures, noting the decline of the former and the growth of the latter. His second dimension was horizonal integration noting the growth of multi-institutional systems 'and consequent shift in the locus of control from community boards to regional and health care corporations'. The third dimension was the extent of diversification, noting the growth of 'polycorporate' and conglomerate enterprises, sometimes with both profit and not-for-profit subsidiaries. His fourth dimension was vertical integration, noting the shift from single level of care to multiple level of care facilities. His fifth and final dimension was industrial concentration, in which he noted 'the increasing concentration of ownership and control of health services in regional markets and the national as a whole'.

The other (equity) concept of distributive efficiency relates to what any given observer considers to be distributive justice. In the health field for instance this might consist of a policy statement that more resources ought to be devoted to caring for the elderly as opposed to providing acute medical care, or that the existing geographical distribution of health care or social class distribution of resources was unacceptable. Indeed, all these judgements have been made in respect of Britain. (respectively DHSS 1981 p. 32; DHSS 1976c; and Townsend and Davidson (1983)) Clearly, therefore, distributive efficiency is a value judgement springing from the a priori views of a particular observer about how health care resources ought to be distributed. [1] Lee and Mills note that whilst the economist 'may have little to say about how much redistribution should take place, he can ... help to evaluate the performance of the policies adopted for this purpose, and identify the factors which limit or extend their scope' (1979 p. 39). In summary therefore, the key concept in distributive efficiency is equity: do people receive what are considered by the observer to be their 'needs'? As Tisdell (1982 pp. 389-419) has observed, where the nature of a market prevents the assessment of performance in terms of allocative efficiency, and especially where it is closely controlled by a public body 'an ... approach has been generated

which judges the social acceptability of the
industry's organisation and outcomes. Structural,
behavioural, and performance characteristics are
used as indicators of economic performance.'
    Distributive efficiency seems in fact to be
treated as being of great importance by governments
so far as health care is concerned. One major
approach to this is of course to provide (as do all
three countries covered in the present volume)
resources for better care to those with insufficient
to purchase their own. The distribution policy for
these resources also has an effect, for example the
RAWP arrangements in Britain or the matching funds
between federal and provincial governments in
Canada. Such policies do not always have their
ostensibly intended effect (see Chapter 5 below),
and analysts such as Galbraith (1963) and Starr
(1982) have argued that producer sovereignty can
only be offset by the creation of consumer
institutions of 'countervailing power'. The
creation of organisations such as the British
Community Health Councils (see Chapter 4 below) can
be seen as an attempt to do just this, whilst the
existence of 'not-for-profit' organisations is an
alternative approach.
    At the level of arbitrary judgement,
distributive efficiency is simple to conceptualise:
A should have more of resource X, and B should have
less. However, the building of reasoned arguments
about equity is much more problematic, as one
current controversy will suffice to demonstrate. As
is well known, access to (say) the services of a
general practitioner in Britain is nominally open.
The question arises however as to whether in
practice each socioeconomic group in the population
receives equitable access, or whether, as is
sometimes alleged, the middle classes obtain greater
access. On the face of it, the latter is not the
case, for there is in fact a tendency for
consultation rates to rise with falling social
class. However, if it is assumed that lower social
classes have greater health care needs (due to their
greater morbidity rates), then the higher
consultation rates are not as high as the relative
morbidity rates would suggest that they should be.
On this latter interpretation then, there is inequitable distribution to the poorer socio-economic
groups. (Townsend and Davidson 1983 pp. 77-8)

DYNAMIC EFFICIENCY

The concept of dynamic efficiency is concerned with the identification of the optimum rate of technological change within an organisation. (Shepherd 1979 pp. 7-8) Its concern is with the relationship between investments and costs, and with the means of optimising future benefits derived from current investment. From the point of view of an organisation which is considering major investment in new technology, the important questions concern the timing of the purchase and the costs and benefits (to the organisation) likely to be consequent upon the adoption of the technology.

Considerations of dynamic efficiency seem not yet to have become current in the public sector, nor are there many examples of academic studies relating it to health care within Britain. In the USA, however, policy initiatives such as Certificate of Needs Legislation have been used in an attempt to control the costs of new technologies. (Joskow 1981) However, a number of points can be made about its application to this field. Firstly, the pace of technological development is now very rapid and involves some very large sums of money indeed (Perrin 1978). This makes the concept of dynamic efficiency _prima facie_ applicable to health care technology.

Secondly, the timing of purchases can have a considerable effect on both price and benefits derived. Since manufacturers' total costs of development and production will tend initially to rise and costs per unit will only later fall as the learning curve is ascended and output volumes increase, and since early years of production will often be protected by patents from competition, initial pricing strategies are likely to take the form of premium pricing. (Cooper 1966) Typically therefore, prices will fall in due course with the onset of competition. It might also be hypothesised that later production will have corrected early design faults. An estimate will also need to be made of the expected period over which benefits will accrue, and of an appropriate discount rate. (Bierman and Schmidt 1984)

Thirdly, it is certainly the case, that a number of unsought consequences (in terms of costs) have followed from the introduction of technology without sufficient prior analysis. These are well documented in the monograph 'Expensive Medical Techniques'. (Council for Science and Society 1982 pp. 18-20) This notes that expensive medical techniques usually 'turn up first as a cuckoo in an unsuspecting (health authority's) nest'. Examples include the apparently routine replacement of, say, an X-ray machine with the next generation of machine which is capable of performing more advanced tests, the appointment of a new Consultant with a special interest which has financial consequences that have not been thought through, the presentation by local voluntary fundraising organisations of a piece of equipment (such as a CT scanner) without any contribution to running costs, and the situation where a health authority is pressured into funding on a routine basis a service originally started on outside research funds. In all these cases, there is little opportunity for managers either to plan the timing of a technique's introduction or to assess its full financial consequences. (See also Altman and Blendon 1979)

MANAGERIAL EFFICIENCY

The concept of managerial efficiency (often referred to as X-efficiency) refers to internal organisational performance (Leibenstein 1956) rather than the intraorganisation behaviour which is the focus of allocative efficiency. Managerial efficiency may be defined as the ratio of inputs to outputs; inputs may be expressed in physical terms (known as technical efficiency) or in terms of money. (Lipsey 1966 p. 231) [2] It should be noted that the concept is a relative one, implying that there are at least two sets of figures for comparison; comparisons may be over time, across organisations, or, as is discussed below, between different methods. Economic theory predicts that perfect competition would result in complete allocative efficiency, but the absence of such competition means that organisations are able to focus more narrowly on internal efficiency (often ignoring externalities, that is costs not borne by the organisation). Managerial efficiency is therefore a less radical concept than allocative efficiency, since it is not concerned with whether some organisational activity is worth carrying out at all, but only with the least cost means of provision.
    One approach to managerial efficiency, cost-effectiveness analysis, '... involves the prior setting of goals and attempts to ascertain the

programme capable of achieving those goals at minimum cost or, alternatively, the programme which will maximise the goals for a given cost'. (Lee and Mills 1979 p. 39) [3] Hence the steps in cost-effectiveness analysis are as follows. Firstly, the desired objective(s) must be defined, in terms which are capable of being quantified. Secondly, at least two alternative methods of achieving the objective must be identified: for instance Klarman et al (1973) studied the relative efficiency of hospital dialysis, home dialysis, and transplantation in increasing survival after kidney failure. Thirdly, the respective costs of each alternative must be assessed, as fourthly must the respective benefits of each; benefits of alternative programmes must of course be measured in the same terms. Finally, the ratio of cost to achievement for each alternative can then be compared and a choice made. Discussion now turns to exploration of some of the data requirements and difficulties associated with this process.

Objectives of a programme must be defined in a way which allows it to be observed whether and when they have been achieved: the link with the concepts of effectiveness discussed in Chapter 2 is plain. Examples from the health field might include years of survival after the onset of a particular disease or the reduction of the incidence of a particular disease in the population. Ostensible goals such as WHO's 'Health for All by the Year 2000' are best seen as mobilising slogans to inspire action. One problem with defining objectives is that there is a temptation to define them in proximate terms such as increasing the percentage of a particular diseased population who receive a particular treatment; in such an example, analysis would focus upon different organisational arrangements for delivering that particular treatment. But built in to such an analysis is the assumption that the treatment is worth giving. No doubt this is probable in many cases, such as increasing the coverage of vaccination and immunisation, but as Cochrane (1972) and Chapter 2 above have noted, the field of health care is characterised by lack of knowledge about the effectiveness of many of its programmes. [4] This temptation to choose proximate rather than ultimate goals is compounded by the general reluctance of actors in organisations to think in terms of goals at all (see Chapter 5 below).

Data requirements for the costing of programmes are discussed in more detail in the next section, but three points can be made here. Firstly, any item which is not included in the costings will be treated by managers as a 'free good' and its use maximised. Hence in Britain, health authorities were able to achieve apparent efficiency improvements in the use of pharmaceuticals by reducing the amount of hospital prescribing by 'shunting' the cost onto the open-ended budget for general practitioner prescribing. Secondly, the question arises as to whether externalities or social costs not borne by the organisation should enter into the calculus; economic theory suggests that they should (Lee and Mills 1979 p. 37), but the incentive within an organisation whose budget is finite must be to ignore them. Hence in practice travelling time and cost for patients and relatives is often treated as a free good. Thirdly, if the costs of alternative programmes occur at different times discounting will have to be applied.

Benefits must be measured in the same 'currency' as the objectives. This can create difficulties where a treatment transpires to produce benefits in addition to those which were formulated in the objectives. Klarman et al (1973) found that kidney transplantation both improved survival (the objective) and gave a greater quality of life; since transplantation was best in both respects the study had no difficulty in reaching a conclusion, but if quality of life after transplantation had been poorer, some kind of trade off calculation would have had to be made. It should also be noted that the selection of proxy measurements of performance can create perverse incentives. The use of (say) perinatal mortality rates as an overall measure of health service performance might well encourage managers to devote disproportionate resources to obstetric care, at the expense of other client groups. (cf Blau 1955) Finally, it is an implication of cost-effectiveness analysis that data will be available concerning how far objectives are being attained; in practice health service statistics are often of the 'process' rather than 'outcome' variety thus compounding the temptation to set objectives in terms of services delivered to patients rather than outcomes achieved. The steps involved in cost-effectiveness are summarised in Table 3.2. The following sections examine the techniques involved in the determination of efficiency within a health care organisation.

Efficiency in Health Care

Table 3.2: Steps in Cost-Effectiveness Analysis

1. Define the programme for evaluation in terms of the required objectives, together with the intended measures of success or failure.

2. Specifiy the alternative methods of achieving the programme objectives.

3. Lay out the resource requirements of each alternative and cost them in one of these ways:

   a Economist's Technique
   . Count the cash flows of each alternative, noting them as they enter/leave the organisation:
   . Add the opportunity costs of using those resources:
   . Include the 'externalities', whilst ignoring sunk costs.

   b Accountant's Methodology
   . Count the cash flows of each alternative, noting them as they enter/leave the organisation's accounting system:
   . Include all the non-cash accounting costs where they impact on any external subsidies, grants or taxes.

4. Discount the cash flows and costs at the estimated cost of capital.

5. Count the degree of effectiveness of each alternative method.

6. Compare the ratios of cost to effectiveness for each alternative method.

   This technique usually supplies a 'least internal cost' solution. (See Mooney et al 1980)

METHODOLOGIES FOR COSTING

Costs may be recorded within two alternative systems of collation by two major methods of collection, as

68

illustrated in Figure 3.1. Costs are recorded for a
cost object, be it a patient, disease, or clinician
(in a process known as 'job' costing, where the
actual costs created by the cost object are
collected together): or alternatively on a
specialty, ward, or department (in a process known
as process costing, where the costs associated with

Figure 3.1: Alternative Costing Systems

	Marginal	Total
Job (Patient, Disease, Clinician)		
Process (Specialty, Ward, Department)		

the overall cost area are averaged between the cost
objects associated with that area). Thus 'job'
costing attempts to collect accurate actual costs,
whilst 'process' costing averages total costs
amongst a grouping. 'Process' costing is generally
less expensive than 'job' costing, but the
difference in the quality of the information
provided for decision making purposes is
substantially lower at operating management level.
It has been argued that process costing suits policy
level decision making. (Tomkins 1983; Collville
1982; Anthony and Herzlinger 1975)
    Whichever method of collection is used, the
system of collating those costs can be either a
total costing system or a marginal system. A
marginal costing system does not allocate
'overhead' costs, rather it attempts to collate
costs into cost reports which are traced to a cost
object or cost area. Costs which are not traceable
to one of these, and/or which cannot be
varied at operating management's discretion are
excluded. A total costing system will attempt to
collate and apply all costs into cost reports.
Thus a cost may be allocated to a cost report
using a basis for apportionment which reflects
past practice, rather than current economic costs.
(Horngren 1977) It is interesting to note that a
study by Magee and Osmolski (1979) of medical

specialty costing systems revealved that 35% of
total costs could not be directly traced to
specialties, and thus remained for allocation. This
35% of cost is included in a total costing report,
but excluded from a marginal costing report.
Further, it is likely that with disease, patient, or
individual clinician costing systems, the percentage
of untraceable costs would rise, since some costs
traceable to a specialty could not be further
traced. (See Babson 1973; Piachaud and Weddell
1972)

There is considerable disagreement over these
alternatives, and their respective costs and
benefits. A simplistic summary of these debates
would be to suggest that the marginal costing system
using a job costing collection method produces
information most relevant to operational management
decision making, whilst the total/process
alternative is least suitable, ceteris paribus.
However, it is not possible to say that the
total/process alternative disables management or
that the cost of the marginal/job alternative is
exceeded by the improvements in managerial
efficiency. Since it is difficult to relate process
costings to specific objectives, they will often not
be usable for cost-benefit or cost-effectiveness
analysis, though they can be used for such exercises
as straightforward comparisons of managerial
efficiency over time. The next section is concerned
with the system that accepts costs and communicates
them to management.

METHODOLOGIES FOR ACCOUNTING

All accounting systems record the cost data provided
by the costing system, and report on them. The
costs are recorded after they have been recognised,
and should be the actual historical costs. This is
immediately in conflict with economic theory which
requires that sunk costs be ignored in the short
run, that opportunity costs be included and that all
social costs be recognised. Historical accounts
reflect only sunk costs, exclude opportunity costs
and ignore externalities, concentrating on one of
the following alternative accounting methodologies.
Firstly, there are cash accounting systems.
These record costs only when cash flows result from
an activity. They ignore any changes in indebted-
ness and any loss of asset values. In the British
public sector they are the basis of the cash limit

system, and in the USA it is recommended
practice to maintain a record of 'Sources and
Application of Funds'. (Buckley, Buckley and Plank
1980 p. 134)

Secondly, there are income and expenditure
accounting systems, in which the changes in debtors
and creditors are recorded in addition to the cash
flows into and out of the organisation. Currently
this approach is the basis for all government
department accounting in Britain, and thus the NHS
uses it for its final year end accounting reports.
It is not generally used within the USA outside the
not-profit private institutions.

Thirdly, there are obligation/commitment
accounting systems. These extend the Income and
Expenditure type of system by attempting to record
and report on the management area responsible for
placing orders, as well as cash flows and indebt-
edness. This type of system is currently being
developed and adopted within the NHS. It is also
widely used in publicly controlled health care
facilities in the USA, where it is common for it to
be used with a separate form of accounting (asset
accounting) which is not commonly used in the NHS.

Asset accounting notes the initial cost of any
fixed assets, and attempts to record their subsequent changes in value over time. Depreciation is
the accountant's term for the loss in value of a
fixed asset over a period (generally a year) of its
life. It is an attempt to reflect the loss in value
of that asset caused by increasing age, general
wear and tear, and changes in the assets value on
the market. Assets may be valued historically, at
current (market) value, or at the cost of replacement. In whatever way they are valued, their
'costs' as applied to accounts are not cash costs,
but rather attempts to assess costs using judgements
and standard formulae. They are the accountant's
method of supplying an indication of the costs of
using an asset, and are sometimes treated as representing the opportunity cost of the asset in the
long term. Asset accounting is therefore irrelevant
to the marginal cost reports upon which short run
operating management decisions are often based.

Finally, there are accrual accounting systems.
In these, all costs are applied to the centres
responsible for consuming resources. It is the most
complex system to install, but is best for
integrating cost information for operating
management by emphasising the identity of the
economic unit consuming the resources. The other

systems may partially collect data on resource usage, but can often use a cruder method, for example, recording a cost against the identity which places the order, whilst ignoring that the resource made available is passed on. Accrual accounting should minimise the 'free good' problem associated with other accounting systems. It is required by the Securities and Exchange Commission and therefore is used by larger for-profit health care facilities in the USA. It is also recommended for adoption by not-for-profit facilities. (see Anthony and Herzlinger 1975)

Table 3.3 illustrates how three of the above systems,when applied to the same data in a not-for-profit organisation, can produce considerably divergent results. [5] Additional implications for the assessment of efficiency in an organisation are that the incentives inherent in the adoption of one or other kind of accounting system need to be considered. For instance, accrual accounting treats unused stocks as 'free goods', creating a disincentive to reduce the real costs of large inventories, whilst income and expenditure accounting creates no incentive to seek the most favourable credit terms. The next section introduces the different budget systems that accounting systems report into. Costing and accounting both generally assume the existence of a 'rational economic manager' (see Chapter 5) who will automatically make correct decisions when provided with relevant accurate and timely information. Budget systems are based on the assumption that managers will perform efficiently when a suitable motivational system is applied.

METHODOLOGIES FOR BUDGETTING

All the accounting and costing methodologies discussed above are concerned with recording past events and the actual costs that have resulted. Economic theory, however, requires information on the future, as well as the past. Actual historical costs are indicative of the future and extrapolation of these can provide a useful guide. Budgets are the key tool used to control operating management, and should consist of a statement of intended resource usage, matched to a planned service provision, all stated in financial terms. The financial terms used for this statement of intent are known as standard costs. The name implies their use; they

Table 3.3: A Comparison of Accounting Methods: Cash Accounting, Income and Expenditure Accounting, and Accrual Accounting

Assumptions: The organisation's financial year ends on March 31. A particular consignment of supplies is delivered in February, consumed in March, and paid for in April.

Cash Accounts	Income and Expenditure Accounts	Accrual Accounts
The cost is recognised and charged to the accounts when the payment is made, in April.	The costs is recognised and charged at the time of receipt of the supplies, when the debt is created, in February.	The cost is recognised as a debt in February, and recorded as a cost against the 'consumer' departments in March.

It should be noted that if an organisation uses both cash accounts and income and expenditure accounts, its annual summaries will differ by the size of the changes in debtors/creditors over the year.

If the organisation begins to take 60 days credit during a year, which was not taken last year, and that 25% of all expenditure is on supplies, then the difference between the two will be $\frac{60}{365} \times 25\% = 4\%$.

Thus the annual cash accounts report will differ from the annual income and expenditure accounts report by 4%, with implications for the internal budgetting system. Those organisations which maintain any two of those accounting systems often have an elaborate end-of-year reconciliation system to balance the separate reports.

are the standard against which what occurs will be compared. Thus three distinct stages in budgets can be identified: firstly, managements preparation of and commitment to a plan; secondly, a statement of the standard costs; and thirdly, a comparison of the standard costs with the actual costs achieved. Budgets are intended as a tool to inform, control, and motivate operating management towards efficiency. Budgets specifically designed to encourage managerial efficiency are known as management budgets, or operating budgets, or responsibility budgets, though other terms may be applied. However labelled, the intention is that the budgets should be borne by those managers who control the variable costs of service provision. Information theory can be applied to define the content and timing of information which must be supplied to managers and to produced an information system that meets these needs. (see Austin 1979)

There are broadly two forms of budgets, fixed and flexible, that can be applied to suit two forms of income streams, pre-payment (or prospective) funding, and post-payment (or retrospective) funding, as illustrated in Figure 3.2.

Figure 3.2: Alternative Budget Systems

	Fixed	Flexible
Pre-Payment (Prospective)		
Post-Payment (Retrospective)		

Where a health care facility is supplied with an income stream which is agreed in advance, it enjoys the certain knowledge of its total income (for example, the NHS and Veterans' hospitals in the USA). If the health care facility is paid after supplying a service for the work actually done, its future income stream is uncertain (for example, in establishments funded by fee income). The difference between the two types of income streams has major implications for budgetting and financial control arrangements. Pre-payment systems have proven advantages for the funding agency (generally for government) by setting a limit on annual expenditure. By separting the income stream to a health care facility from the actual workload achieved, a major operational dysfunction is created, since either the facility will suffer an excess of expenditures over income as a result of higher than expected volumes of work, or a low volume of work will encourage expenditure unrelated to current levels of demand.

Flexible budgets are created within health care facilities by use of an internal charging system reflecting the costs of each activity. Flexible budgets relate volume of work achieved to cash inflows paid. The charges payable are often agreed in advance by central formulae, such as Diagnostic Related Groups in the United States. The economist's preference for marginal cost pricing is never applied in its pure form, for accounting systems cannot produce the continuously varying marginal cost of each single addition of health care provided. At best a two stage curve can be used, with a breakpoint set at an agreed volume, as illustrated in Figure 3.3.

Figure 3.3: Marginal Cost Budgetting

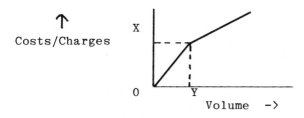

In this approach the charges agreed, OX, cover the costs of low volume (OY) facilities whilst higher volume facilities can receive lower incomes to reflect their greater economies of scale. Clearly the slope of the curve and the breakpoint, if any, are in practice key points for negotiation. It is important to note that a flexible budget implies no limit to total earnings, though it is often suggested that it should. (Ingram 1980 pp. 365-374)

Fixed budgets are also negotiated in advance, though it is the total expenditure which is agreed and not the charges payable. Thus the health care facility can organise itself for the maximum service provision within this previously fixed limit.

Most, if not all, health care facilities enjoy both types of income stream and can provide a mixture of fixed and flexible budgets. The key points of concern to managers involve their joint impact on management actions and any dysfunctional interrelationships. Fixed budgets encourage managers to spend up to the limit, and to keep reserves which are either spent at the end of a financial year or transferable to the next year's budget. Efficiency savings, or underspendings are seen as bad things, for they may trigger a cut in next year's budget. Flexible budgets encourage end of year expenditure too, but do not necessarily motivate managers to minimise costs. Depending on the market arrangements and cost structures they can either maximise volume or income, or minimise cost. This latter point depends on management's ability to restrict either demands upon the facility or access to treatments via increasing queue lengths.

An example may help to reveal a dysfunctional interrelationship. A teaching hospital may receive research monies, agreed in advance; centrally funded capital grants, agreed in advance; payments for work completed in treatment of patients; payments from students for training received; and monies from investment funds. Some of these income streams will be known in advance, and some are subject to uncertainty and will vary over time. It is possible to base the budget system on the uncertain income stream, but it is more general to base it on centres of responsibility. Thus a head of department may be subject to either a fixed or a flexible budgetting arrangement. If it is a fixed budget, the variable costs and incomes can disable any attempt at meeting the set expenditure level. If it is a flexible budget, the department head will have difficulty controlling expenditure on research. A general result is a system that attempts to 'square a circle', with flexibility in a fixed budget and rigidity in a flexible budget.

The issue of budgetary control raises the problem of integrating clinicians into the management budgetting arrangements. The extent of such involvement of clinicians in the financial management of a health care facility varies from country to country. In the USA, common practice is to inform clinicians of their costs for personal income (pricing) purposes, or for the prospective reimbursement process (such as through Diagnostic Related Groups). This of course occurs in a context where if a clinician increases throughput, there is an increase in income with no limit either for the individual or the facility. Hence, cost control systems are designed to keep costs below income at the margin: that is the additional cost and income

resulting from one more patient. This is entirely
consistent with recommended economic practice. (See
Mooney 1983)

In Britain, by contrast, there is as yet no
approved regular system that supplies cost reports
on clinical activity, though some experiments are
currently being conducted (for a summary of these,
see Wickings 1983); clinician involvement has
otherwise been limited to the memebership of one
hospital Consultant (elected by his or her
colleagues) on each District Management Team. This
occurs in a context where the income stream to
health care facilities are fixed in advance and
without reference to the actual workload achieved in
practice, a system which emphasises total costs and
the need to hold expenditure below the fixed income
limit. (See Brooks 1984)

As a result of these differences, the conflict
between medical ethics and financial constraints
differs in the two countries. In the USA, a
patient's inability to pay (for treatment or
insurance cover) can conflict with a clinician's
judgement of need, whereas in Britian it is the
limited availability of total resources for health
care which may conflict with the clinician's
judgement of need. The result is a rationing system
based on price in the USA and on queues in Britain.

It can be seen therefore that budgetting, like
accounting, systems, are likely to have an effect on
managerial efficiency through the behavioural
incentives which they provide. As noted, these
incentives will depend on the precise system of
budgetting adopted, and a full exposition of the
possibilities is not attempted here. However, it
can be noted that issues for consideration would
include potential incentives to managers for saving
on total costs and/or reducing unit costs, rules for
'virement', or the balance of flexibility within
budgets and flexibility between budgets and whether
marginal costing should underlie budgets in order to
concentrate managerial attention on the effect of
varying 'production' levels. Clearly, none of these
issues can be decided without consideration of their
relationship with the type of income stream which
the agency or institution as a whole receives from
its funding sources; this too will create a set of
incentives within the organisation, amusingly but
accurately parodied by Neuhauser (1983) in respect
of Diagnostic Related Groups in the USA.

CONCLUSION

It will be clear from all that has been said above that there is no general agreement about the nature of efficiency. This can best be summarised by drawing attention to four kinds of contrast.

Firstly, the economist and the accountant, just two of the disciplines most readily thought of as having a concern with efficiency, tend to take quite different approaches to the concept. These differences are summarised in Table 3.4. But perhaps the most significant of them is the

Table 3.4: The Economist versus The Accountant

Economist	Accountant
Uses explicit economic theory:	Concentrates on methodology, costing systems and methods, accounting systems and methods:
Proactive: concerned with future economic events, ignoring sunk costs and including all opportunity costs and externalities:	Reactive: collects historical data to report on past events, including sunk costs and generally avoiding opportunity costs and externalities:
Extrapolation: generally derives cost data from statistical methods such as regression:	Interpolation: records all transactions in an account of the business in process or completed:
Prescriptive Audits: audits are conducted and checked for accuracy in comparison with the model's predictions:	Descriptive Audits: audits are conducted mainly to check the factual accuracy of the historical descriptions:
Generally uses ad hoc studies and a variety of methods.	The accountant generally uses routine studies, and methods.

treatment of social costs or externalities; the economist's concern with social and opportunity costs, and the accountant's with a particular organisation's historical costs.

Secondly, there is an important contrast between cost-benefit and cost-effectiveness analysis. The former might be considered to take a longer and wider view, and to be concerned with ultimate ends, whilst the latter takes a narrower and often shorter view, being more concerned with means. Nevertheless it is through such techniques that effectiveness can be linked with efficiency.

Thirdly, there is a major philosophical difference underlying the contrast between allocative and distributive efficiency. Allocative efficiency implies a 'want-regarding' (Fishkin 1979) view of interests, that is, that the consumer knows best. Distributive efficiency assumes an 'ideal-regarding' view, that is that the provider knows best. This question of whose views of health services should count is discussed in Chapter 4 below.

Fourthly, that attention may, in some parts of the health sector, shift away from allocative and distributive efficiency and towards dynamic efficiency. The apparently inexorable spread of high-cost, short-life new technology raises doubts about management ability to date to choose when to leave old technologies and enter new ones.

In conclusion, these differences suggest that consciously achieved progress towards increasing the efficiency of health services will involve two essentials. The first of these is an explicit confrontation of what kind of efficiency is to be sought; this is a value judgement. The second is the involvement in this process of all the professional disciplines which have a part to play in defining the broader concept of health service performance: epidemiologists, clinicians, economists and accountants, as well as those who have a major stake in the behaviour of health services organisations – the public.

NOTES

1. Although it is occasionally denied, the other notions of efficiency considered in this Chapter also carry value judgements implicit in them. Thus allocative efficiency implies that benefits to society as a whole, rather than to a particular section of society ought to be maximised. Managerial efficiency implies that externalities are

Efficiency in Health Care

unimportant enough to disregard.
    2. Technical efficiency should not be confused
with the much narrower notion of engineering
efficiency. The latter refers (say) to the
percentage of potential energy in a fuel which is
actually produced as power by an engine; only one
input is considered, whereas technical efficiency is
concerned with all inputs. (Lipsey 1966 p. 232)
    3. Improved efficiency (that is lower unit
costs) will therefore only result in a reduction of
total costs when a lower than current cost limit is
set, within which objectives are to be maximised.
In the field of health care this can be illustrated
by considering costs per inpatient case. When
efficiency is improved by increasing throughout
(lowering lengths of stay), cost per case will fall,
all other things being equal. However, total costs
will rise as more cases are seen because certain
(for example surgical) costs occur irrespective of
length of stay.
    4. The results of faulty assumptions about
cause and effect relationships are further discussed
in Chapter 5.
    5. For further discussion, see Ingram (1980
pp. 27-39).

Chapter 4

ACCEPTABILITY IN AN EFFECTIVENESS AND EFFICIENCY
CLIMATE

Jack Hallas

INTRODUCTION

The professionals working within Health Services in
the developed world have now become well accustomed
to an organisational climate where effectiveness and
efficiency are constant features of the day-to-day
weather. To some extent, the public has also become
acclimatised to such considerations dominating the
health service scene. Indeed, these two words carry
within themselves a comforting sense of certainty,
of rational objectives, a capability for decisions
to be assessed in numerical terms, and an
organisational sense of direction.

The intent of this Chapter is to cloud the
issues addressed in this book by suggesting that
there are dangers in too closely considering health
services in such terms. It will cast a necessarily
brief glance at the differing understandings of the
word 'acceptability' held by relevant health service
actors. Amongst this cast of thousands are
professionals, especially those in the medical
arena; the Members of corporate public bodies, such
as Regional Health Authorities and Community Health
Councils in Britain; and lastly, and least, the
academic laity.

At its simplest, this Chapter can be seen as
merely a gloss on the familiar concept of 'Inputs –
Outputs – Outcomes'. Organisations, whatever their
reason for existing, are largely if not
overwhelmingly concerned with their inputs and
outputs. The refreshingly naive assumption that it
is comparatively easy to adopt such concerns, and
readily apply them to all organisations, has been a
feature of central policy directives in Britain for
some years now. (NHS Management Inquiry 1983 p. 13)
After a period in the mid-1970s when the cry was

that the NHS was becoming over-politicised, the current policy tendencies of central government are now directed to setting the boundaries of debate in terms of economic and business considerations. What does become obscured in such an organisational climate is the necessity to consider more closely the outcomes of decisions based on internal efficiency and the corporately rational assessment of what constitutes effectiveness.

At a more complex level this Chapter is also concerned with justifying subjectivity as a means of assessing the acceptability of the outcomes of decisions largely based on criteria assumed to be objective. To take an analogy from physics, it can be said that the NHS is organisationally still living in a philosophically Cartesian world, with Newtonian explanations holding good for the middle ground. In the realms of the infinitely small and the infinitely large, such explanations do not hold. At the point where an individual meets a doctor or nurse in one of the millions of transactions being carried out daily in health services, indeterminacy takes over its explanatory role. When considering the NHS as a feature of the universe of social activities in the UK these relativistic explanations carry most conviction. The latter part of this Chapter will return to this theme, but as it is always prudent to move to the complex from the simple it is necessary in the first instance to return to more mundane considerations.

The Collins Dictionary (1980) definition of 'acceptable' reads as follows: 'acceptable: 1) satisfactory, adequate; 2) pleasing, welcome; 3) tolerable - acceptability or acceptableness; (n) ...' It is the third definition of 'acceptable' that is given greatest weight throughout this Chapter. The satisfactory, adequate, pleasing, and even welcome, can emerge in any climate - witness the English summer - but a cold climate can often be more vigorous and stimulating. For polemical purposes the 'via negativa' of what is perceived as intolerable will not be far below the surface in certain sections of what follows.

Polemic is very often parochial. A Weltanschauung might have suited Schopenhauer, but for academic scramblers in the foothills an attempt to range over the acceptability of health resources from professional and public perspectives in a variety of cultures is a subject apt for the Proustian scale. The latinists had a phrase commended to the reader, 'mutatis mutandis'; if

readers in the USA can link the material in this
Chapter to Federal initiatives and directives on
such issues as renal dialysis, and states' funding
of Medicaid, then they can congratulate themselves
on their ingenuity. The social and cultural
differences that exist, for instance, between the
USA and Britain are particularly apparent when
considering the acceptability of health care
provision in these countries. What would be totally
unacceptable in the USA, for instance a nine-month
delay in obtaining 'cold' surgery attention, would
in Britain be viewed as normal and acceptable.
Whilst not forgetting these cultural differences, it
is now time to examine some aspects of professional
attitudes to acceptability where professionalism
often papers over the cultural cracks or gulfs that
exist socially.

PROFESSIONALISM AND ACCEPTABILITY

It is easiest to start with the medical profession
working within large units in the NHS, thereby
unfortunately having to exclude General
Practitioners from consideration, and look at some
of their attitudes towards professional
acceptability. This is not to say that nurses,
administrators and all the other professionals
working within the organisation do not have similar
concerns, but after all the founding fathers of the
NHS did see it as essentially a medical service.
Furthermore, the medical profession is not only the
most powerful so-called cohesive body within the
NHS; it has also agonised more publicly than most
about ethical considerations that necessarily entail
acceptability as a major factor.
        It is assumed in any consideration of the work
of doctors that they are doing their best for their
individual clients. Another given is that there is
no chance of improving the quality of life if no
life exists, so the saving of life comes before all
other considerations. Already one edge into an area
of debate. In recent years in Britain the increased
publicity given to heart transplant operations has
been a subject of controversy within the medical
profession. What is often seen by the outsider as
heroic surgery is rated as unacceptable by some
clinicians. Those most closely involved respond by
pointing out that they are merely building on
existing medical knowledge, and responsibly carrying
forward the resultant expertise and thereby

extending the life chances of individuals. In the NHS context, and this activity can take place nowhere else in Britain at the present time, there are organisational considerations that also have to be brought into the debate. What proportion of resources should be devoted to this activity, and how should those resources be distributed? Quickly, then, the question of acceptability comes to focus on the concept of organisational triage. Originally 'triage' was a military device to maximise the effectiveness and efficiency of fighting forces, by sorting out casualties into priorities for treatment, and often more importantly for the individual fighting man, non- treatment. When treating life's casualties, if the NHS is to be perceived as a 'repair shop for the nation' (Kaprio 1983) then there comes a point where certain bodies are considered as beyond repair, and consigned to that great scrapyard in the sky. In his thought-provoking book, 'Triage and Justice', Winslow (1982) heightens a debate on social justice by focusing on life-saving medical resources. More pertinent to this text are his comments on the ethics of utilitarianism and egalitarianism. Health organisations' considerations of scarcity of resources on a macro scale often assume the Benthamite slogan of the greatest good for the greatest number as a normally acceptable criterion for policy decisions on the allocation and distribution of scarce resources.

It is at this point that acceptability carries different meanings for some NHS clinicians and the organisation they work in. Until recently, the NHS was a monopsony employer of medical labour; there was nowhere else to go. In Britain in the late 1970s and early '80s, thanks largely to the ideological endeavours of a Socialist government (Klein 1980), the possibility of working in the private sector became more of a reality. This would have enabled those clinicians with an individualistic ethic and similar professional expertise and inclinations to move over full-time into smaller health organisations, where the individual user of services is of paramount importance. Ethics had less to do with some of those clinicians who saw and seized the opportunity to work both within the NHS and within the private health sector; it had more to do with enhanced earnings. Sadly for these expectations, the private health sector in Britain seems to have plateaued, if not even declined somewhat from the rosy expectations of growth entertained some years ago. The move from a parasitic growth of private health care practice feeding on the body of the NHS to a symbiotic relationship of mutual benefit to both parties has therefore to be seen as a possibility for the future. So, for now, the conflict of interest between clinicians in the NHS and the policy-makers at central and local level concerned with increased effectiveness and efficiency will not be reduced by the existence of a large 'private practice' bolt hole for some of the members of one of the parties involved. Authorities will constantly encounter medical professionals saying that their proposals or decisions are professionally unacceptable. As in most instances, there will be a negotiating process, trimming of sails, and at any cost an avoidance of serious conflict; the boundaries of the acceptable and unacceptable will constantly shift. What safeguards exist to prevent the unacceptable, through an incremental growth of custom and convention, becoming the acceptable, or at least tolerable, perhaps even satisfactory?

Peer review is, or is supposed to be, such a safeguard. Before establishing the sanctity of such procedures it would be as well to hear the Devil's Advocate. 'We are not answerable to our peers, because each of us knows that were we to shoot a patient straight between the eyes, we would be hard put to it to find a colleague who would not reassure us that it was all for the best, that anyone would have done the same, that the patient was asking for it anyway, that if it hadn't been us someone else would have done it for sure, and that the patient's really better off now.' (Hart 1983) This is a powerful expression of day-to-day informal review, which might be better described as a particular example of working class solidarity. Nevertheless, the suspicion remains that even in formal peer review procedures there is an element of professional banding together which can never be totally discounted. Very rarely does the public become aware of individual clinicians' unaccountable practices reaching such a pitch that their peer group refuses to work with them until they mend their ways, or insists on them being placed in a position where they can do least harm. Such extreme cases do exist and in not inconsiderable numbers, and are dealt with within the organisational NHS with varying degrees of rigour.

In Britain since 1974 the individuals most immediately concerned with bringing together the differing perceptions of acceptability held by doctors and authorities have been the representatives of clinicians and General Practitioners on District Management Teams. (DHSS 1972) In management terminology, this is a 'non-job'. They are part-time, as against four full-time professional officer members of the team. A recurring theme is that they have constantly to maintain a precarious balance between being seen as a traitor to the medical profession by giving in too easily to managerial pressures or, on the other hand, being seen as a hero by not giving an inch and standing firm on grounds of professional propriety. It is no wonder that over the last decade, in common parlance, the definition of it as 'coronary country' has taken root, nor that the rotation of incumbents has often been rapid. But if the current emphasis on effectiveness and efficiency is maintained then it becomes crucial, from the perspective of acceptability, to establish a strong countervailing force concerned with constantly defining and, if necessary, redefining the boundaries of what constitutes normal and acceptable practice. At local level the 'Cogwheel' Medical Divisions which exist, with varying degrees of viability, in the hospital setting could more easily assume a role of acceptability watchdogs. As the Griffiths Report (NHS Management Inquiry 1983) recommends for very different reasons, the divisions would need strengthening by administrative support, and to have a remit from the Health Authority which enjoined them regularly to review the outcomes of policy intiatives in the light of professional acceptability. This modest proposal would allow for an element of recognition that the three-fold process of considering proposals under the headings of inputs - outputs - outcomes took place formally and routinely at a crucial point within the hospital organisation. It would also allow for a degree of peer review that was not concerned with the unacceptable behaviour of individuals, but was seen as an advisory body on professional attitudes, particularly where effectiveness and efficiency initiatives were concerned.

This section began with a referral to the hightly dramatic debate on heart transplantations. This is a topic where acceptability in a professional sense is particularly relevant. It is not the only example. In the next section reference is made to other crucial issues concerning medical treatment, necessarily from other perspectives.

Acceptability

Now it is time to turn to other aspects of
acceptability, taking as an example a Regional
Health Authority in England which, for a number of
conflicting reasons, brought into the glaring light
of day questions of professional and lay attitudes
to acceptability that capture many of its aspects
when linked to effectiveness and efficiency.

THE OXFORD REGION STORY

Since the Reorganisation of the National Health
Service in 1974 many hard decisions have been taken
in the interests of increasing organisational
efficiency in the service. Under the Labour
Government of May 1974 – May 1979 closures of small
hospitals and reduction of services, e.g., casualty
units in Inner London, were officially described as
the consequences of a programme aimed at
rationalising existing services. From mid-1979 to
date the rhetoric has changed. Now the rationale
for closures and reduction in services has been
couched in terms of stressing urgent economic or
financial necessity as being a main consideration.
Whatever the rhetoric, the impact of these changes
in service were spread over time and dispersed
nationwide. Localised concern about the
acceptability of these decisions existed from time
to time in varying degrees of intensity, as
witnessed by the reports of numerous Community
Health Councils. But the process was successfully
conducted by creeping decrementalism. In September
1982 the Oxford Region's Team of Officers produced a
consultative document entitled 'Implications for the
Oxford Region of Current Government Policy – A Paper
for Information, Discussion and Consultation in the
Oxford Region'. For the first time there was
initiated a national debate on the consequnces of a
drive for effectiveness and efficiency based on a
wide-ranging assessment of possible outcomes, and
one worthy of quotation in extenso. The following
extracts from the consultative document pick up the
major features of the paper after an introductory
sections concerned with the financial position of
the Oxford Region:

    This Region is no longer is a position to
    provide services comprehensively .... In these
    circumstances ... new ways in which services
    and resources can be matched must be considered.
    Broad options are:

87

1. the steady reduction of levels of service to the value of several million pounds each year could be continued as it has during the last 2-3 years and by a process of gradual erosion the service could be diminished and the financial books balanced. The disadvantages of this method are related to the low morale which results from repeated arbitrary cost-saving exercises and the choice of inappropriate services for cuts.

2. a single very radical reduction of services could be made in one year in order to create a central reserve which could be redeployed according to, say, a five year plan, releasing the service from the annual burden of making cuts and giving the appearance at least of some agreed developments taking place. This is difficult to effect in a situation where the service is under great pressure and the initial savings would be taken from areas of undoubted patient need. On the other hand, this approach would restore some stability and sense of progress to the service, albeit at a reduced level.

3. a replanning of the pattern of services could be undertaken with the emphasis on cheaper methods of delivery of care. Many desirable elements of the service would have to be abandoned and some of the costs borne by patients, but the essential quality to individuals in need could be maintained.

Recognising that any revision of health services resulting from these measures would have the effect of establishing different, lower standards of services in the Region from elsewhere in the country, it is suggested that a combination of options 2 and 3 might be employed, option 1 being regarded as no longer acceptable or even workable. The NHS principle of equality of opportunity for or even access to services would certainly be broached for the first time.

The Government Minister concerned with the 1982 Ministerial Review, which triggered off the debate, had written in a letter to the Regional Chairman that 'these are hard decisions and the considered choices inevitably rest with the Region. However, the realities of our present resource situation demand that some sort of fresh assessment be made.' The Regional Team of Officers (RTO) took him at his word, and produced some urgent strategic approaches for discussion and consideration which hit the national media weeks later in October 1982. The Minister must have felt like the minister of religion who prayed for rain, and when rewarded with a deluge said 'Lord, we prayed for rain, but this is ridiculous'. Just some of the 'fresh approaches' included:

a) a period of residence qualification for eligibility for non-emergency services;
b) rationing treatment and care among the elderly;
c) reduction in the distribution of Accident and Emergency Departments;
d) a rationing system for investigative procedures;
e) some services, e.g., cold surgery, family planning, completely abandoned;
f) a much greater responsibility on families or voluntary services to provide transport, laundry, food and some personal 'hotel' services;
g) creating public awareness of lessened opportunites for health care.

Not all the Oxford Region's Team of Officers propositions have been listed above, nor have the more 'far-out' ideas been deliberately selected. What is clear is that thinking the unthinkable and listing the unacceptable concentrated the mind wonderfully. Just as it is easier within an organisation to detect what is not 'value for money', a glib current slogan much in vogue, rather than what constitutes value for money, so it also becomes easier to define the acceptable, or tolerable, by listing the unacceptable. In the pursuit of efficiency one easy strategy, often adopted, is to shift the burden on to another party by 'cost shunting'. An example of this ploy is that stated in f) above. Now it is not unreasonable in some developing countries for a population to accept that they must find their own way to hospital and that kith and kin should provide food, some laundry, and play a part in 'waiting on' the patient. It is often in the light of custom that practices are considered acceptable or unacceptable. To overturn or seriously disturb custom is perilous process, either for a government or for a powerful organisation. The proposition listed as g) above went on to suggest that General Practitioners and Community Health Councils could play a part in re-educating the public to accept a new pattern of use. Like most educational processes this would take a considerable time to achieve, especially if taken in hand at a time of massive reduction in services previously enjoyed as of right. Neither would the workers employed in the ambulance service or the domiciliary and catering services readily accept wholesale redundancies as anything else than a dismantling of the NHS. On the other hand creeping decrementalism, if financial circumstances permit, could move in the direction of shunting these costs without seriously bringing into question public and worker acceptability. For example, ambulance services in many parts of the UK have reduced the use of vehicles for non-urgent cases to a greater extent than was the case three or more years ago. The NHS strikes of 1982, when ambulance workers withdrew their labour, helped this process by demonstrating that inpatients and outpatients could find their way to hospital by other means if they were forced to do so. Apart from blatant injustices which cry out for redress, minor adjustments of custom are often a painless way of achieving efficiencies. This would suggest that linking efficiency with urgency is a mistake from a perspective that considered acceptability as a necessary criterion.

Another strategy for achieving an appearance of efficiency is to stop doing something. Proposition e), to abandon some services within the Oxford Region, with the examples given of cold surgery and family planning, takes one into this area. It is unthinkable that cold surgery would not be done by anyone, so the paper goes on to suggest, surely tongue in cheek, that the private sector would presumably take it on. Cold surgery has, in England, waiting lists which would be considered totally unacceptable in the USA. Perhaps in the NHS one is still living peaceably because of the British tolerance of, and indeed liking for, orderly queues. This is one example of where there is a similarity of views that exists amongst users of the NHS and the customers, clients, or consumers, call them what one will, of private health care. Their tactics differ, however. The private sector is built on a foundation of immediate or appropriately timely response to clients' and doctors' perceived

needs.   Rather   than   queue-jumping   it   is   a   similar
situation   to   a   theatre   that   has   seats   available   in
the   more   expensive   parts   of   the   house,   but   if   you
cannot   afford   them   then   you   must   queue   for   the
cheaper   seats.   An   abandonment   of   cold   surgery   would
result   in   a   flood   of   clients   that   the   private   sector
in   Oxfordshire,   or   indeed   in   England,   could   not   cope
with.   To   end   this   meditation   on   totally
unacceptable   propositions,   and   tongue   in   cheek
again,   if   such   an   eventuality   did   come   to   pass   it
might   prove   necessary   to   call   in   experts   from   the
public   sector   to   advise   the   Secretary   of   State   how
he   should   encourage   the   private   sector   to   take   a
leaf   out   of   the   NHS   book.

The   effectiveness   of   provided   services   has   not
been   forgotten,   but   it   is   necessary   to   consider   just
one   more   consequence   for   the   users   of   NHS   facilities
that   necessarily   follows   from   a   drive   towards
effectiveness   and   efficiency;   that   is   a   greatly
increased   use   of   overt   and   covert   rationing.
Proposals   a),   b),   and   c)   would   certainly   be   overt
rationing,   and   d)   would   be   a   more   disguised   form   of
the   same   principle.   Special   circumstances,
particularly   the   existence   of   a   rapidly   growing   'new
town'   at   Milton   Keynes,   led   the   RTO   to   suggest   a
residence   qualification   for   eligibility   for   non-
emergency   services.   Their   paper   remarks   that   this
is   a   commonly   adopted   practice   of   housing
authorities   and   that   the   NHS   allows   referral   back   to
place   of   origin.   The   analogy   of   course   (like   most
analogies)   does   not   hold,   but   as   an   example   of
lateral   thinking   it   displays   some   ingenuity.   The
elderly   are   always   present,   and   especially   in
developed   countries   the   elderly   elderly.   A   DHSS
report   (DHSS   1981a)   gave   an   insight   into   the   extent
to   which   the   population   of   England   and   Wales   aged
over   75   was   taking   up   resources   in   the   acute   sector.
In   their   paper   the   RTO   asked   how   can   treatment   and
care   of   the   elderly   be   rationed?   The   easy   answer   is
to   institute   a   more   rigorous   system   of
organisational   triage.   Finally,   in   terms   of   overt
rationing,   a   reduction   in   the   distribution   of
Accident   and   Emergency   centres   would   be   the   most
public   manifestation   of   a   dramatic   and   drastic
reduction   in   services.   More   covertly,   a   rationing
system   for   investigative   procedures   could   take
advantage   of   user   ignorance   or,   in   Rudolf   Klein's
term   'idiot   consumers',   to   allow   professionals   to
clear   the   acceptability   barriers   easily.   As   an
internal   response   to   necessary   cost-cutting   in   the
name   of   efficiency,   this   is   already   an   increasingly

common practice in the NHS today.

PUBLIC BODIES AND OTHER RESPONSES

So, in terms of acceptability, what was the response of the public as represented by Community Health Councils in Oxfordshire to this 'information, discussion and consultation paper' prepared by officers of the Region? The Chairman of the Oxford RHA was in no doubt about his perceptions: 'The document provoked a thoroughly worthwhile debate about the future of the health service in this region and has given the authority a valuable indication of what professionals in the service and the consumers of the services want to see in future. The response has been widespread, interesting and constructive. It's been one of the most successful public consultation exercises we have had .... In my view they represent a programme for action which will help this Region to continue to provide the excellent service for which it is well known, in a period of severe financial difficulty.' (Roberts 1983) No uncertain sound of the trumpet here.

As might be expected, the perspective of the Community Health Councils (CHCs) was rather different. The Oxford City CHC hastily arranged a public meeting, which took place about a month after the publication of the consultative paper. In spite of foul weather, some 120 members of the public gathered together to voice their concerns. Voluntary bodies and agencies were represented but did not show a very high profile. Political activists, in groups and as individuals, certainly made themselves heard, as did those present who were health service workers. An observer calculated that NHS staff were a 'noticeable' constituency at the meeting. Whether one views this presence as a cynic or an idealist is a matter of individual propensity. At the end of the evening the meeting passed overwhelmingly the following resolution:

> That this meeting reaffirms its belief in the principles of the National Health Service: that is the provision of a comprehensive health service free at the time of need, funded out of general taxation. This meeting urges the Community Health Council to press Oxfordshire Health Authorities, Members of Parliament, the Department of Health and Social Security, and the Secretary of State that resources should be

found to maintain the National Health Service along the lines of its basic principles.'

The CHC for Oxford wrote to the Chairman of the Regional Health Authority on 1 November and set out its initial response to the consultation paper. In general terms this initial stance was as follows:

The duty of a Community Health Council according to the establishing legislation, 1973-74, is 'to represent the interests in the health service of the public in its district ....'

The National Health Service was established by the 1946 Act to provide a complete medical service, free of charge at the time it is required, for every citizen. It is therefore the duty of CHCs to defend this concept, work for improvements in health services and contribute towards making the NHS a comprehensive preventative and treatment service, as envisaged by its founders.

Many of the propositions outlined by the RHA Paper would meet the outright opposition of this CHC to the full extent of its capacities. These would include any system of rationing by age, sex, nationality, locality, etc.

Some of the ideas in the Paper would warrant further examination should additional information be forthcoming. These would include widening the range of day surgery, and the re-centralisation of specialist support to GPs.

However, this CHC believes that some of the RHA's financial troubles can be laid at its own door and some of them could be rectified even at this late stage. To be specific:

1. Failure to establish a proper system of allocating money to the districts.
2. Failure to ensure overall supervision of the way money is spent by District Health Authorities and Family Practitioner Committees.
3. Failure to further a programme of National Health Service land sales.
4. Failure to introduce a management structure

which provides accountability for services and finance.
5. Failure to monitor services and involve Community Health Councils and all National Health Service Staff in efficiency programmes.

In January of the following year the Chairman of the CHC issued a press statement. After rehearsing the points given above, it stated that no adequate reply had been received from the Regional Health Authority, either from the Chairman or the Regional Team of Officers. At its meeting in this same month the Regional Health Authority Members did a deal of back-pedalling. They were advised that 'no services can be identified which can be totally abandoned by the NHS'. The Regional Strategic Plan was to be urgently revised with a target date of some nine months ahead. There should be in this strategy a commitment to a much greater emphasis on community care with a lesser dependence on institutional-based (and therefore capital-dependent) services. The reduction of Accident and Emergency Departments was not considered feasible. There had also to be more means found for 'rewarding' efficiency and providing incentives.

Given this 'pushing back' of the target date for a regional strategy, the steam was taken out of the public pressure for information about what was really going on behind the scenes at the regional level. The impact of public opinion on this revisionist stance is hard to assess. All the members of the Authority had received copies of the CHC's letter and statements. The media at local and, to a much lesser extent, national level had had their say. In terms of formal consultation with representatives of the general public, to those nearest to this aspect, the consultation was derisory. At all times the RHA had emphasised that there had been a 'major consultation exercise' for some three months after publication of the original 'consultation' paper. Noticeably in its subsequent statements (Oxford RHA 1984), the RHA referred to its taking into account government policies and priorities, and the way in which it had drawn on the skill and experience of doctors, nurses, administrators and other specialists throughout the Region. Also, in their preface to the summary of the outline proposals for the development of health service in the Oxford Region 1984-1994, they were quite straightfacedly reporting that the last year

(1983) had seen much discussion about the future of health care. In spite of all the comments made by Community Health Councils throughout the region, there was not even a mention of their part in this 'process of consultation'.

'A NEW WAY FORWARD'

It is worth looking in some detail at the summary of the long term proposals of the Oxford Regional Health Authority in the light of the themes of this book. Their strategy is succinctly set out in the document published by them in June 1984. (Oxford RHA n.d. p. 3) The cornerstone of the new strategy is to be a campaign covering all aspects of health care provision and disease prevention with a particularly vigorous thrust at cancer and heart disease. Interestingly enough, the first stated aim is to reduce the demand for treatment, a most powerful means of appearing to increase efficiency, and secondly to promote a healthier lifestyle for everyone, which is effectiveness operating at a supreme level. The growing tendency for the public to resort to 'do-it-yourself' activities in many aspects of their social life gives weight to this cornerstone, but there must be some doubts about the foundations.

By chance a community physician based in Oxford, years ago, meditated on some of the factors which must be borne in mind when considering the mounting of healtheducation campaigns. (Muir Gray 1977) The whole article well repays reading closely, but just one of his themes is particularly relevant in this context. How, he asks, can one interest a whole population in modifying their behaviour to receive benefits in health and pocket, which will only become apparent in some distant future, when the bulk of them are paid weekly and seek instant gratification based on a 'Monday to Friday' mentality? Since he wrote, the boom in home ownership has reduced the impact of' weekly rent' as a factor in his argument. But, on the other hand, the massive increase in credit card usage, and the increase of earned or enforced leisure, which can reduce time horizons to 'what shall I do today', add new dimensions to his perspective. Implicit in his line of thinking is the not unprofitable approach to this topic taken by the 'Black Report'. (Townsend and Davidson 1982) Crudely put, there are two nations involved, the upper and middle social classes, and

the lower social classes. A trap frequently fallen
into by middle class planners is for them to assume
that their desiderata, for example long-term
benefits, privacy, and health bestowing prudence,
are shared by the whole population, and only need an
injection of 'vigorous campaigning' to stimulate a
massive response. In this arena effectiveness and
efficiency must bow to acceptability; colloquially,
you can lead a horse in the direction of water, but
you can't force it to drink.

Next in the document is 'sharing care'. It is
thought that if the Oxford Region joins forces more
effectively with local government authorities and
voluntary organisations, it can do more for people
by spending more money better and by spending it
together. To many local authority councillors and
officers this siren song will sound suspiciously
like an invitation to have costs shunted onto
their shoulders. How far the 'sharing care' approach
has been accepted by local authorities is not
clearly stated in the body of the document. There
is an acknowledgement that the RHA accepts that
local authorities are no better off than the health
service, but what the state of play is at present is
hinted at by the comments that local authorities
reactions were being sought to some ideas for
working together to improve care for the elderly;
local authorities could expand health promotion
roles; and for the elderly mentally infirm Local
Authorities should provide a wide range of services.
In spite of a protestation by the RHA that repeated
references to more care in the community are not
aimed at shifting the burden of care onto local
authorities, the fact remains that there is a
massive barrier of acceptability to overcome. A
common weakness of organisational drives for
effectiveness and efficiency is induced
isolationism. There are many autonomous features of
the current plan which are wholly under the control
of the Regional and District Health Authorites. A
just criticism of the 'old' Regional plan was that
it was a self-regarding exercise. Given that this
'new' plan gives an air of excitement to a different
way of looking at the total provision of health care
to a large population, initial informed judgements
on the plan would have been helped had some
indication been given that this excitement is shared
by those invited to share. A week may be a long
time in politics, and politicians dislike the
academic tendency to have long memories. Although
the original statement of intent, referred to at the

start of the case study, to reduce or abandon
services may have worked well on the minds of
government ministers, recollections of that document
at local authority level might well increase
suspicions that injure the RHA's credibility.
Indeed, effectiveness and efficiency can increase
the level of credibility to some observers of the
scene, but unless there is a conscious seeking for,
and checking out of, the amount of acceptability
that these new initiatives have to other interested
parties, then credibility can soon be lost, and on a
significant scale that needs bridge-building of a
high order to remedy.

In a highly professional organisation, which
any health service in the western world must be,
voluntary effort is usually seen as peripheral, at
best symbiotic and at worst parasitic in its
relationship to the health care system. It will
need a considerable indoctrinal effort to modify
these attitudes at all levels within the medical and
nursing professions. Oxford RHA perhaps makes a nod
in this direction when the plan acknowledges that
training for all staff will be an important feature
of the implementation of the Regional strategy.
More tangibly, it mentions in the self care and
informal care programmes for action 'To maintain
and, if possible, increase grants to voluntary
bodies,' For services for the mentally ill it
offers 'positive encouragement from health
authorities', and that is about it. When the
document gets down to 'The Strategy in Practice' any
reference to voluntary effort disappears, and one is
left with this major theme: 'the need for
imaginative collaboration with local government
authorities'. If this is 'joining more effectively
with local councils and voluntary organisations'
then other chapters in this book need re-writing in
terms of defining the use of the word
'effectiveness'.

It would take up more space than is merited to
comment too closely on the selling points that the
new plan has in terms of being fast moving and based
on problem solving. Two glancing observations.
Efficiency is often linked with fast moving, but the
terms in this equation are not interchangeable; to
be fast moving does not entail that one is
efficient. One has Karl Popper's word for it that
when one has solved problem (P^1) then one moves
to the problems inherent in the solution as (P^2).
(Popper 1972 p. 244 ff) Even more emphatically he
states how important it is that one has subjected

to critical analysis what (P^1) really is. The seeming lack of seeking such a critique from outside of the members and professional advisers of the NHS in Oxfordshire raises proper doubts as to whether the new plan has got its problem totally right. What reservations, in terms of acceptability, do the mentally ill, mentally handicapped, the elderly and their relatives, have in regard to the end of their dependency on old, large institutions? Instead of the eradication of largeness and the substitution of discrete smallness of organisation Schumacher (1974 p. 201 ff) suggests that the trick is to create 'smallness within largeness', and that in organisational terms this can be a very cost effective exercise.

What must bulk larger in this review is the emphasis placed on 'New Buildings' in the plan. Although declaring that they are not 'hooked to buildings so much' the strategy document states that they will need some new buildings: some to help to change the style of care, some to meet the needs of an increasing population, and some to replace worked out buildings in acute hospital complexes. Also they would want to invest in new buildings which would help in running hospitals more efficiently, on fewer sites.

In an article published in 'The Lancet' the Secretary of the Oxford Community Health Council expressed his personal views on the effect that Oxford city teaching hospitals had on the allocation of financial resources. (Richardson 1984) He remarks that probably the most remarkable achievement of the Oxford Medical School over the past six or more revenue-cutting years was to increase the number of teaching hospitals from two to three, in his words 'a breathtaking example of innate, anonymous, and unaccountable power at work'. He estimates that had the teaching hospitals' costs in 1981/82 been held to the same proportion of total expenditure as in 1978/79 some £2.7 million would have been available elsewhere in the service. More starkly put, during this four year period other parts of the NHS were deprived of several million pounds in order that the teaching hospitals might evolve and expand. 'Under the Banyan Tree of the Oxford teaching hospitals nothing much else seems to grow ... and many services struggle even to survive'. Finally he comments that what is needed is management that is accountable to, and enters into discussion with, the general public about what is needed by way of prevention, treatment, and care.

In its outline strategy the Regional Health Authority expresses concern about the availability of acute medical and surgical beds, and the problems of 'fitting in' teaching alongside the rapid pace of treatment. It states that the Region and District Health Authorities and the University are working together to develop a strategy to help with this problem. A high expertise in problem solving will be required, because in the section on 'Money' it is noted that if they are to develop the priority services (mentally ill, mentally handicapped, and the elderly) it will mean that acute services must become 'even more efficient'. In terms of development money, over the next ten years, the acute sector, under the new dispensation, would be some 8% worse off in terms of increased expenditure in comparison with a 'status quo'. So perhaps the Banyan Tree is in for some pruning; but it is a sturdy growth, and can almost miraculously put out new branches.

Oxford Region's average length of stay figures are, even now, very low. In 1982 'general medicine' showed an all England average length of stay of 10.7 days. In Oxford the 1983 average was 8.4 days. In trauma and orthopaedics the national average was 12.5 days, in Oxford 8.7 days. Any drive for more efficiency in this context would rapidly increase the already reported distress of some patients over early discharge from hospital. (Richardson 1984) In terms of acceptability there also need to be considered the professional responses of nurses and doctors to a working environment based on such rapid turnovers. The increased emphasis on day care contained in the plan offers to these professionals, and the public, the proposition that a quarter of all acute cases should be treated as day cases. In the context of the triad of efficiency , effectiveness, and acceptability, it would be encouraging to know that the general public was fully aware of this significant change in time spans of hospitalisation. The plan states that day care would be cheaper, make fuller use of facilities, and, given proper selection of suitable patients would cause little extra burden on community services. Its aim is to transform short stay patients on to a day patient basis - not to seek additional cases. The Oxford Region plan thus offers a sizeable rapid repair shop facility for NHS patients in the acute sector. This is a significant change in approach that above all demands the education of the public that the original 1982 paper suggested could be undertaken by General Practitioners and Community Health Councils. Somebody must do it, otherwise the public might consider that they were being 'short changed' as tax payers, and that the trend towards this type of development was unacceptable. Thus in shaping the pattern of new buildings over the next ten years the Region faces the unenviable task of bringing into line its objectives with those of the various District Health Authorities, whilst retaining credibility with the government of the day, and representatives of the population. So what, at the time of writing, are the early omens?

In early June 1984 the Minister for Health met with the Chairmen of the District Health Authorities in the Oxford Region to discuss their long term plans for developing health services. He was quoted as saying that he welcomed the broad aims of the strategy that had been put out. (Clarke 1984) It was in line with the Government's determination to modernise the service to the public and the buildings from which that service is provided. No problems seem to arise from that quarter. However, in early July 1984 members of the Regional Health Authority had to run a gauntlet of public protesters before their monthly meeting. During the meeting, which is statutorily open to the public, they had to cope with a barrage of comments and abuse from the public gallery. (Hyde 1984) At the time the Community Health Council was making its submissions to the Regional Health Authority. Back in the late Autumn of 1982, members of the major health service unions and other activist groups had set-up a 'Who Cares' campaign. All through 1983 they monitored the progress of the Regional Health Authority whilst it was drawing up the outline strategy document. Their basic opposition was succinctly summed up by one protester at the meeting as 'the myth of community care' which they regarded as just another name for cuts, closures and job losses. Their suspicions exploded into anger at the Regional Health Authority meeting and a level of personal abuse which is not worthy of quotation was directed at the Chairman and Officers. The CHC had not been involved with the 'Who Cares' campaign to any extent. Although having some sympathy with the message of the campaigners their medium of personalised abuse was unacceptable, and, in the opinion of their Secretary, counter-productive. During the meeting the Chairman said that he had met representatives of the 'Who Cares' campaign to discuss the document, and that a full reply to their comments had been sent out that day.

In England it still causes a _frisson_ when the full panoply of an Authority's meeting is interrupted by the strangled cries of the general public, although the incidence of such events has grown since 1982, principally at District levels. This public confrontation is reported here not to shock the more genteel reader, or outrage the upholders of dignified public life, but to indicate a fundamental problem for authorities that arises when their rationales for radical change are overtly based, either wholly or partly, on efficiency and effectiveness criteria. The excitement engendered at the top of the organisation arises from redefining ways of doing things; it is the 'challenge of change'. At lower levels in the organisation, as piecemeal information filters through, this excitement is transmuted into sullen resentment about possible changes in the status quo ante that they are powerless to resist openly. The result is that middle managers in the organisation are ground between the upper and nether millstones of pressure from the top to speed the process of change and a significant increase in often covert inertia from the bottom. (Schon 1971) This is a common feature of working life in the United Kingdom, but not, one gathers, in Japanese organisations. (Goldsmith 1984) Perhaps there is a self sacrificial aspect of Japanese culture which, when linked up with organisational survival, results in an eager willingness to adapt readily to radical changes in working practices. This is not so apparent in Britain. Here, one man's efficiency is another man's redundancy; there, the contract between management and worker is, in the larger organisations, expressed in terms of a lifetime's commitment by both parties. What might be transferable is the willingness of Japanese top management to create forums for workers at all levels to express their views on ways to introduce new practices that are an aid in furthering efficiency within the organisation. It would be unfortunate if the anger expressed by representatives of many health workers in the Oxford Region at the meeting reported above was perceived as having been contained and possibly dissipated. Paradoxically, effectiveness and efficiency within organisations are perceived in terms of concentrating on productivity, with a certain impatience of consultation, or 'jaw jaw' sessions;

in practice far more discussion of acceptable
alternatives has to take place at many more levels
within the organisation if real progress is to be
made by a willing, or less unwilling workforce.

These comments on a public document are
deliberately biased. They demonstrate a partial
view, they are subjective. The Oxford Strategy has
vision, it is an honest attempt to re-order a
pattern of health care provision perceived in the
1980s as suitable for the 1990s. All are good
things, as is the high degree of professional
competence displayed in the detailed, full
documentation underlying the summary discussed
above. So why so much jaundiced comment? Those who
accept the following quotation as containing a
fundamental truth will know why: 'Man's capacity for
justice makes democracy possible, but man's
inclination to injustice makes democracy necessary.'
(Niebuhr 1945) Those who do not are in the
position of the earnest enquirer who asked jazz
pianist 'Fats' Waller 'What is rhythm'. His reply
echoes down the years: 'Lady, if you got to ask, you
ain't never going to have it'.

There is another gulf that exists between the
perceptions of authorities and those concerned with
representing the views of the public at large. If
the collective experience of CHCs since their
inception in 1974 is examined it becomes clear that
there is no such thing as a general public or whole
population that is actively aware of, and concerned
about, the wide range of health service issues that
exists at any one time. (Hallas 1976) There are
many publics with specific interests. Amongst these
specific interests there are three issues which
constantly recur on CHC agendas. There are strong
loyalties for smallish local hospitals, which can
offer human-scale services; accessibility of
services, including transportation problems in rural
areas; and the level of services provided for the
elderly, the mentally ill, and mothers and children.
From Community Health Councils' reports it would
seem that acceptability is often measured by what
their members can see, touch, smell, and tick off on
a watch. Typical and frequent comments can be
encapsulated as

> The hospital was clean, comfortable and had a
> pleasant atmosphere;

> It is difficult to find your way to the clinic,
> and the bus service is bad;

Acceptability

> There are long delays in the Outpatient
> Department;
>
> The kitchen was hygienic and cooking smells
> were kept to a minimum;
>
> Geriatric patients were woken up and put to bed
> at unreasonable times:

and so on, often <u>ad infinitum</u>. This is the very
stuff and substance of what constitutes
acceptability in the minds of users of services. If
there is a 'general public' view of the NHS it
resides in services being perceived by them as
proximate, expeditious and non-intimidating. Too
great a concentration on organisational
effectiveness and efficiency tends to drive out, or
reduce in importance, consideration being given to
these factors. Of course the overwhelmingly
acceptable outcome for a member of the general
public is that they are made well, improved, or at
least not made worse by the attentions of the NHS.
Where the impact of effectiveness and efficiency is
specifically understood as increasing the chances of
such outcomes then there is no contest. Where the
issue is more complex, as in this Oxford experience,
then the expression of public opinion of
acceptability labours under certain difficulties.
Nothing could be more proximate than being treated
at home. Day surgery units are certainly
expeditious. A clinic should be less intimidating
than a high rise District General Hospital complex.
Nevertheless the underlying suspicions of bodies
representing the public, whether they be the 'Who
Cares' group, the Community Health Council,
voluntary bodies or the media, remain. They are
concerned about the massive shift of resources, not
in terms of whole populations of users and workers,
but in personalist touches such as, what might
happen to eighty year old Mary Smith, and what could
happen to fifty year old porter John Doe? The short
answer is that nobody knows. Mary might die, John
might be pleased to get hold of some ready cash by
receiving a redundancy lump sum. But unless health
organisations make an attempt to personalise their
public pronouncements, and demonstrate that they
have a realistic awareness of possible unfortunate
outcomes for individual users of their services, and
all levels of their staff, they will do nothing to
lessen this gulf. 'In Search of Excellence', the
managerial gospel for today has much to commend it,

not least when it equates organisational success
with a policy of getting close to the customer.
(Peters and Waterman 1982) How one gets close,
managerially, to users of the NHS is a problem for
the future, not tackled so far by the Oxford
Regional Health Authority. They are not alone. The
drive towards rapid improvements in effectiveness
and efficiency within the health service necessarily
results in a tendency to push consideration of
possible unfortunate outcomes into the background.

SOME FINAL COMMENTS

This Chapter is an imperfect gloss on the triad:
Inputs - Outputs - Outcomes. The point, and the
difficulty, of any form of trinitarian thinking is
that all three aspects must be given equal attention
simultaneously, and given equal weight. This is
difficult. An easy way to close would be to echo
G.K. Chesterton and say that the world is perfectly
rational, but not quite. Effectiveness and efficincy
are perfectly rational, but not quite. Having a
sense that the reader who has persevered thus far
deserves something more learned, the last words will
be left to one of the seminal thinkers of this
century. Michael Polanyi delivered the Terry
Lectures at Yale University in 1962. In them he
demonstrated that commitment to a cause can be
better understood when it is recognised that we all
know more than we can tell. (Polanyi 1966) What
constitutes 'efficiency' in the tacit dimension
might, for instance, be an unspoken wish to retain
established, measurable relationships, than being
able to prove that improvements have been made. This
could result in a distaste for and explicit resistance to radical innovations. 'Effectiveness' might
be a tacit assumption that if everybody worked as
well and as hard as oneself, then a more effective
organisation would inevitably be the result.
'Acceptability', as a slogan, might rest in a tacit
belief that all authority is to be distrusted, in
any person, at any time, and in any place. We can
never expect total explicitness. What we do know,
and can act upon, is that reasoned explicit dissent,
if timely and listened to, can reduce avoidable
mistakes. Let Polanyi have the last word '...to
know that a statement is true is to know more than
we can tell, ... we commit ourselves to a belief in
all the as yet undisclosed, perhaps as yet
unthinkable consequences.' (1966 p. 23)

Chapter 5

PERSPECTIVES ON IMPLEMENTATION

Stephen Harrison

What is implementation? The syntax in which the
term generally occurs suggests a quite
straightforward notion; as Pressman and
Wildavsky (1979 p. xix) note, as the derivative from
a verb it must govern some objective such as
'policy', 'plan', or 'programme'. The implication
is of a pre-existing decision, which is subsequently
put into operation; one World Health Organisation
(WHO) document (1981 p. 7) notes that 'programmes
have to be brought to life'. A second
characteristic of this notion of implementation
is that it is a relatively straightforward
and technical organisational activity (Pressman
and Wildavsky 1979 p. 143). This characteristic
has been manifest in both academic treatments of
public administration and management, and in the
formal structure of work organisations. Thus the
criteria and processes of decision making are
conventionally regarded as central to the
management task (Drucker 1979 p. 314) or even
synonymous with it (Simon 1957 pp. 2-3), and public
authority members, boards of directors or
trustees, and corporate managers are seen as
determining policies which are handed for
implementation to more junior organisational
levels.
     Within the last fifteen years, however,
developments have occurred which challenge the
notion of implementation as logically and
pragmatically subordinate to decision making or
policy making. Firstly, there has been an
increasing realisation that implementation is not
unproblematic; a number of studies, perhaps the most
seminal of which is Pressman and Wildavsky's (1979)
examination of project to provide jobs for minority
groups through the economic development of Oakland,

California, highlighted the incidence of implementation 'failure'. Secondly, there has been an increasing acceptance of the need to pay more attention to alternative theoretical perspectives on organisations (which as Hall and Quinn (1983) note are often both the intended means and intended objectives of policy, as well as comprising the milieux in which policies are determined) and decision making. Some of these theoretical perspectives suggest that the policy implementation distinction is not a valid one, thereby raising questions about what is meant by 'unsuccessful implementation'. The overarching purpose of the present Chapter is to put forward perspectives aimed at assisting the critical examination of the events reported in Chapters 6, 7, and 8, and in framing the conclusions set out in Chapter 9. The following section attempts to characterise some relevant theories of organisation and decision making along lines relevant to the notion of implementation; as Rohrbaugh (1983 p. 279) has noted 'it is essential that our methods of organisational analysis reflect diverse and competing values'. The next four sections deal more fully with the types of theory identified in the preceding section, and illustrate them with relevant material from the literature. The penultimate section considers the general applicability of such theories to health services organisation, whilst the final section raises a number of questions to be explored in the empirical material of subsequent Chapters.

TOWARDS A TYPOLOGY OF THEORIES

A wide range of theories, from a wide range of academic disciplines, has been developed in order to explain and/or guide the behaviour (especially decision making behaviour) of managers and other actors in work organisations. Hall and Quinn (1983 p. 282) have noted the need to integrate the similarities between subfields of social science, and it is not surprising that there have been numerous attempts to classify these theories, one of the most recent and best examples being that of Pfeffer (1982). The classification of theories for general teaching purposes will always be problematic since such theories have a range of content and it is not self-evident which of this should be used to structure them. The present purpose is, however, more modest and it is only necessary to choose

dimensions which are relevant to the concept of
implementation. This of course results in the joint
classification of theories which have many
dissimilarities and it needs to be clearly
understood that a shared categorisation of a number
of theories does not imply that they are similar in
all important respects, nor indeed that theories
which are not categorised together are completely
contradictory. Two dimensions of classification are
employed, as follows.

Firstly, a distinction is made between on the
one hand those categories which assume that
rationality can be seen or sought at the macro
level, that is organisational level, and, on the
other hand, those which assert that rationality
can only be seen at the micro level, that is amongst
groups, occupations, and individuals. This roughly
corresponds to Ham and Hill's (1984 p. 96 ff)
distinction between 'top-down' and 'bottom-up'
approaches. Viewed at the macro level, the
organisation is a 'tool with the ultimate goals of
accomplishing its tasks and acquiring
resources.' (Rohrbaugh 1983 p. 268) At the micro
level it is a collection of groups and individuals
about which it is necessary to ask the questions
'whose goals, whose policy, whose objectives, whose
problems?'

The second distinction which is made concerns
the extent to which actors are assumed to seek to
maximise their objectives. On the one hand, there
are theories which assume that analysis and value
judgements precede action, which is in turn aimed
at maximising the attainment of one or more
objectives: in other words, proactive behaviour. By
contrast, other theories assert that such a model
places too great a burden on human inclinations and
cognitive abilities and makes heroic assumptions
about how worthwhile at the margin is further
information and analysis in the production of better
results. This second kind of theory therefore
substitutes for the notion of 'maximising' that of
'satisficing' (Simon 1959) the assumption that
actors are primarily reactive (to problems), and
that the tendency is for them to adopt the first
reasonable solution which presents itself, rather
than to search for a best solution. A matrix (see
Figure 5.1) can be constructed from those two
dimensions, to give four types of theory; a label
has been attached to each of the four types, which
are now discussed in turn.

Perspectives on Implementation

Figure 5.1: A Typology of Theories

	Rationality at Macro Level	Rationality at Micro Level
Maximising/ Proactive	Unitary Models Models	Pluralistic Models
Satisficing/ Reactive	External Control Models	Bounded Rational Models

UNITARY MODELS

The defining features of unitary models are firstly
that it makes sense to speak of 'organisational
objectives' [1] and secondly, that processes within
organisations can, or should be seen as part of a
logical sequence of objective-setting, followed by
more detailed planning and policy making, the
assembly of the required resources, the execution or
implementaton of the plans, and finally a monitoring
or evaluative process. In some theories, the
process is seen as a feedback loop, with the
possible modification of plans or objectives as a
result of the evaluation process. Thus rationality
is seen as relating to the macro level, and
behaviour as being (or needing to be) maximising and
proactive.

Unitary models probably comprise the largest
and most pervasive category of theories about
organisations for perhaps three reasons. Firstly,
such models have a long history; the founding
fathers of both academic and applied theoretical
work in organisations espoused them. Thus Weber
(1947 p. 337), notwithstanding the tendency of later
commentators to underestimate the subtlety of his
views, did believe that bureaucracy, characterised
by formalised values and rules, offered potentially
the most efficient type of organisation. Other
management or administration theorists, such as
Fayol (1971 p. 20 ff), stressed the necessity for
unity of direction, the subordination of individual
interests to organisational interests, and
maximisation of output through job specialisation.
Secondly, unitary models have found expression in
the work of a wide range of academic disciplines; as
Allen (1979 p. 109) notes, they are a basic

108

assumption of micro-economic theories of the firm, operations research, and quantitative decision theory. Thirdly, some such theories have a technical, impersonal quality which may allow them to be seen as non-threatening. This is especially true of the quantitative theories, and of cybernetic approaches to control in organisations such as that of Beer (1981); the bare essentials of the latter are that control cannot occur without the existence of a clear set of aims, good information about the extent to which actual events correspond to these aims, and a means of correcting any discrepancy between the two.

Relatively few writers (examples are Kahn (1977) and Bakke (1959)) have made the claim that such unitary models approximate to actual behaviour in organisations. On occasions the models are used as 'aunt sallies' to emphasise the divergence between espoused theory and practice (Allen 1979 p. 109) or to aid in the construction of alternative explanations of events. (Allison 1969) More commonly however, the models are used normatively, as an ideal to be aspired to and to guide attempts to improve the performance of organisations. A recent example of this from the health field is WHO's 'Managerial Process for National Health Development' (1981) which conceptualises desirable health services organisation in terms of the model reproduced at Figure 5.2. Models such as this are also easily linked with some versions of systems theories; a recent example from the field of health care is the proceedings of a NATO Conference in which the need to take 'mulitple well co-ordinated actions to reorient service delivery patterns' is consistently stressed. (Pannenborg et al 1984)

What kinds of notions of implementation failure spring from unitary models? The possibilities seem to be three fold: of failure at the objective – setting or planning level, of failure in the transmission of plans to the implementors, or of failure on the part of the implementors. The first of these, failure of the planners, would consist of insufficient analysis of the cause/effect relationships involved in achieving the planned objectives, leading either to non-attainment of objectives, or their attainment at the expense of substantial unsought and perverse consequences. Such mistaken views of the cause/effect relationship can take a number of forms. At its simplest, insufficient time and resources might be allowed for

Figure 5.2: Managerial Process for National Health Development

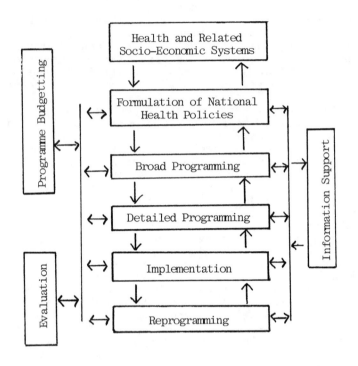

Source:

WHO, Guiding Priniples for the Managerial Process for National Health Development, WHO Geneva, September 1980.

Reproduced by kind permission of WHO

implementation; Gunn (1978) cites British legislation for the control of pollution as a victim of resource starvation. Alternatively, the policy might simply be mistaken in its assumptions about cause and effect; Pressman and Wildavsky (1979 p. 149 ff) observe that employment subsidies would have been much more likely to create jobs than the capital subsidies actually offered in the Oakland Project. Another manifestation of this kind of failure is the perverse consequence; Thompson (1981 p. 255) notes that the payment practices originally used in the US Medicine and Medicaid schemes actually encouraged doctors to invest in expensive equipment and to charge higher fees, whilst Klein (1980 p. 35) notes that the decision of the British Labour government in the mid-1970s to attack the private health sector by phasing out paybeds from National Health Service hospitals might well serve to boost the construction of privately-owned hospitals. Finally, the specification of proxies as measures of the achievement of objectives can also produce perverse consequences as shown in Blau's (1955) famous study of competition within employment agencies which led to wasteful duplication and discrimination against difficult-to-place clients.

Transmission failures are in a sense all failures of communication. Firstly, there is a difficulty in precisely specifying what is to be implemented; vague instructions will not guarantee that the plan is implemented as intended, whilst over-precise specification risks inflexibility, slavish obedience, and goal displacement whereby the rules become an end in themselves. (March and Simon 1959 pp. 37-8) Thompson (1981 p. 254) points out the difficulties which can result from an inability to impose a common language on all those involved in implementation. Secondly, lower level participants in an organisation can see very clearly when their superiors are consciously uncommitted to a policy; Rose (1976 pp. 139-140) shows how US Federal officials' lack of commitment to a management-by-objectives scheme resulted in its divorce from the budgetary process. Thirdly, there are possible failures of coordination, resulting in a programme becoming out of phase or out of balance; as both Pressman and Wildavsky (1979 p. 102 ff) and Thompson (1981 p. 262) have shown, coordination difficulties increase more rapidly than do the number of actors to be coordinated.

Failures on the part of the implementors fall

into two straightforward categories. Firstly, they may be incompetent. Thompson (1981 p. 269) observes that it is rarely possible to recruit staff from scratch for a new programme, and that especially in the public service, career patterns involve personnel in a wide range of generalist tasks over their working lives. Secondly, the implementors may not obey; in terms of unitary theories, this is perversity and is frequently the subject of polemic about 'wreckers' [2] though, as the next section shows, alternative theoretical perspectives lead to different conclusions.

In summary then, unitary models see the implementation process as 'top-down'. Once effective policies have been devised, any implementation failure is a problem of control: the problem of how those formally at the top of an organisation can impose their will. Such notions have been characterised by Majone and Wildavsky (1979 p. 178) as 'implementation-as-control'.

PLURALISTIC MODELS

The defining features of pluralistic models are the assumptions that the organisation consists of individuals and groups (hereafter referred to as actors) who do not necessarily share the same objectives and for whom it provides a context for the maximisation of their own interests. Thus, the focus of rationality is at this group or individual level. A further feature follows from these: that incompatibilities between the objectives, interests, or values of different individuals or groups are mediated through the exercise of power. Differences in relative power (for as Dahl (1963 p. 26) noted, power is a relationship rather than an object) will either be so great as to result in the achievement of one actor's objectives rather than another's, or will not be so great as to result in domination and will instead result in compromise outcomes which are quite different from the intentions of any single actor.

Such pluralistic models of organisations can be divided into three main groups, dependent upon the assumptions which they make about the distribution and exercise of power. Firstly, there are those models which assume that power in societies and organisations is reasonably widely distributed. Such models are often seen as originating from the views of pluralist [3] political scientists such as

Dahl, but have also been used in the analysis of organisations; thus the early writings of Fox (1966 p. 2) refer to organisations as 'miniature democratic states'. The view of power which is taken in such models is that its exercise can only be observed when there is a conflict, indicating that an actor would have behaved differently if allowed to. This, of course, leads to the conclusion that where no conflict is observed no exercise of power has occurred, and that since neither society nor organisations are constantly driven by overt conflict, there is no one dominating social actor.

Secondly, and by contrast, there are 'elitist' models of organisation in which it is assumed that power is distributed cumulatively throughout societies and organisations, being preponderantly held by an elite. Again the origin of such theories may be found in the work of political scientists, in this case Mosca (1939) and Michels (1915). More recent applications of such ideas to organisations have been made by Pfeffer (1981), Allison (1969), and Bachrach and Baratz (1970). The latter authors have also provided an alternative view of power; in addition to being manifest through conflict, power may be exercised in order to prevent conflict through a process of 'non-decision making', or keeping issues off the agenda for action. The views of some sociologists of the professions (Johnson 1972) are consonant with elitist theories.

The third kind of pluralistic theory, human relations theory, whilst accepting that social actors (especially workgroups) have interests of their own, has failed to deal explicitly with the notion of power. This is perhaps because their authors have tended to argue that the nature of such interests, largely in the satisfaction of social needs, made them reconcileable with each other and with management objectives. (Rose 1978 p. 124) [4] As well as their different treatment of power, the various theories make different assertions about what it is that actors seek to maximise. It is of course not necessary to specify this a priori, though some theories do; thus Johnson (1972 p. 39 ff) argues that professionals seek privileged lives and conditions of work, whilst Crozier (1964 p. 170) argues that workgroups seek to maximise their autonomy from other groups.

'Implementation failure' in pluralistic theoretical perspectives can only be usefully considered as the failure of a specified social actor to attain his objectives; such failure could be for any of the reasons already specified within the unitary model. In addition however, implementation failure will be expected to occur where the specified actor is insufficiently powerful in a situation where his objectives run counter to the interests of other actors. (Gunn 1978 p. 174) Thus, failure no longer appears as the result of perversity, but of the rational pursuit by actors of their own legitimate interests.

In this 'political market' actual events are likely to differ from the precise intentions of any single actor. This can occur in at least five different ways. Firstly, distributive policies are likely to succumb to the politics of the 'pork barrel'; as Thompson (1981 p. 261 ff) has noted, this tends to result in all important actors receiving some resources, often therefore insufficient to achieve any result. Secondly, redistributive policies are likely to be particularly difficult to implement; Allen (1983) points out that negative veto power is often more effective than the positive power of direction. Thirdly, increasing the number of actors in a given situation produces not merely the problems of co-ordination already mentioned, but problems of compliance. Pressman and Wildavsky (1979 p. 107) calculated that a programme requiring agreement between different actors at seventy decision points (by no means an exceptionally complex programme) would have less than a 50% probability of success, even if the probability of agreement at every decision point were 99%! [6] Fourthly, the use of apparently objective management techniques does not solve these problems; as Rose (1976 p. 141 ff) pointed out 'management-by-objectives is best invoked for non-political (i.e. non-controversial) concerns of government'. Finally, organisations are likely to be dominated by the concerns of those who work within them, rather than those whom they ostensibly serve; Alford's (1975 p. 190 ff) study of health care in a US city shows it to have been dominated by producer interests at the expense of consumers.

In summary then, the pluralistic notion of implementation shifts its perspective from that of control ('how can we implement this policy?') to one of negotiation and compromise ('what kind of policy is likely to be implementable?'). In this perspective, the ability or inability to implement different options actually determines policy decisions in the first place (Hunter 1984 p. 63). Pluralistic notions of implementation have been summed up by Majone and Wildavsky (1979 p. 180) as 'implementation-as-interaction'.

BOUNDED RATIONAL MODELS

Bounded rational models of organisation share with pluralistic models a focus on the objectives and behaviour of actors below organisational level, but differ on the dimension in assuming that these are reactive in response to perceived problems rather than proactive in pursuit of objectives. The basis of this second assumption is the cognitive incapacity of human beings to fully consider the costs and consequences of all alternative courses of action in pursuit of objectives. Hence, actors react to perceived dissatisfactions with the status quo, and their reactions take forms similar to those of their reactions to previous similar problems.

Much of the above is summed up in the term 'bounded rationality', and the best know exponents of the model have been Simon (1957) and Cyert and March (1963). In summary the work of these theorists views organisations as coalitions of actors, each of whose perspectives on any given 'problem' are likely to differ; in particular, actors in different functional sections of the organisation are likely to see problems in terms of their own function and to seek to apply solutions which rely on their own skills. Due to the cognitive limitations of humans, a focus on the short-run tends to predominate and information is simplified or ignored. The end result of these tendencies is that attention is given to only one or two problems at a time, novel solutions are only attempted when familiar ones have failed, and the pattern of choice of solution is 'satisficing': adoption of the first satisfactory solution rather than search for the optimal solution.

Highly consonant with the work of the bounded rational theorists is the theory of incrementalism, developed by Lindblom (1959 and 1979). The essentials of incrementalism are that decision makers choose activities which are not very different from present ones because of both the cognitive difficulties of evaluating more distant strategies, and the difficulties of implementing them in opposition to the power and interests of those who benefit from the status quo. Hence, policy options are simplified by the deliberate omission of unrealistic objectives and by not attempting to consider all the possible consequences of actions. Actions thus become exploratory, with marginal corrective action being taken when there is dissatisfaction with events. 'Policy' only appears in retrospect as a long chain of amended decisions with no expectation that a problem will ever finally be solved. Moreover, there is a concentration on means rather than ends, and in particular upon the relationships between agencies. (Vickers (1965) The net effect of all this is that organisations change only marginally and spasmodically: hence the term 'disjointed incrementalism'. In short, 'policymakers attack specific problems in the light of the general ... perspective that controls both explanatory hypotheses and the range of solutions that they are willing to consider.' (Lindblom and Cohen 1979 p. 77) Bounded rationality theories are also consonant with role (Kahn et al 1964) and action theories (Silverman 1970 p. 149) to the extent that they focus on actors within organisations and the generation of meanings and expectations through interaction with other actors rather than through independent choice. [6]

One aspect of bounded rationality has been developed by Allison (1969) as a possible explanation of decision making processes. In his 'organisational process paradigm' he observes that the mass of organisational behaviour may well be 'determined by previously established routines'. In other words, the existence of standard operating procedures and the 'parochial priorities' of specific sections of organisations preempts many choices of action. Another aspect of bounded rationality has been developed by Dunsire (1978 p. 152 ff), who makes the point that there are different 'orders of comprehension' at different organisational levels; a superior cannot therefore give implementation instructions to a subordinate until he has confirmed with the subordinate that the instructions are sensible ones to give.

Empirical studies have confirmed at least four major insights of bounded rational theories. Firstly, organisational action tends to be geared to reacting to problems rather than achieving objectives. Rose's study of the US President concluded that 'a President's priorities are set not by the relative importance of a task, but by the relative necessity for him to do it.' (1976 pp. 151-

4) Governments are 'overflowing with objectives.' (Rose 1976 p. 145) Moreover, policy demands are often manufactured inside organisations, for as Brown said of welfare organisations 'most initiatives come from the grass roots - from the desire of people at the point of delivery for developments that would make their own work more useful, interesting or satisfying.' (1975 p. 156) As Hunter summarises it, policy emerges from the combination of discrete operational decisions. 1984a p. 63)

Secondly, the response to a problem involves a drive to action of some kind, irrespective of whether it ameliorates the problem. Pressman and Wildavsky note that policymakers cannot often predict the consequences of their actions, but when there is a clamour for action, any plausible course will suffice (1979 pp. 125-6) to which Rose adds that 'activity is proof of the importance of a public person' (1976 p. 3).

Thirdly, the means-ends logic of the unitary and pluralistic models is contradicted by the evidence, since it is the means rather than the ends which are 'what the action is about.' (Pressman and Wildavsky 1979 p. 98) Duffee and Klofas (1983) point out that means and ends do not necessarily co-vary and that changes in the formal objectives of prisons (from custody to treatment and vice versa) have not resulted in changes in their mode of operation. In addition, there can be solutions searching for problems to attack, a context in which Thompson has placed much of medical care (1981 p. 265). In short, the policy-implementation distinction becomes less valid.

Fourthly, policies tend to be vague enough to allow post facto rationalisation about the success of their implementation (Ham and Hill 1984 pp. 105-6). As Rose (1976 pp. 5 and 135) notes 'a politician who commits himself to a precise objective loses status if he fails', though at the same time both Thompson (1981 p. 258) and Haywood (1983 p. 55) have found that a more precise formulation of parameters can sometimes ensure that outcomes resemble intentions. This process of rationalisation can sometimes extend into the taking of what amounts to symbolic action. Hence Rose (1976 p. 156) and Ham and Hill (1984 pp. 6-7) have referred to the appointment of special advisers or the setting up of a new agency as examples of this phenomenon. This symbolism is often unconscious or unintentional; for instance both Hill (1981) and

Pressman and Wildavsky (1979 p. 146) point out that those who have fought for the creation of particular policy statements often lose interest in their implementation. Brewster et al (1981) distinguish the 'espoused' (formal) policy priorities of an organisation from the 'operational' priorities, that is those which the behaviour of powerful actors indicates to be treated as important: 'the makers of operational policy are rarely aware of it'.

Bounded rational models therefore suggest that the success or failure of implementation should not be judged upon whether formal objectives have been acheived or have been claimed to have been achieved. Rather, the questions should be 'has the policy made things better than they otherwise would have been?', and if so, 'better for whom?'. As Dunsire (1978) puts it 'implementation is in the eye of the beholder'. The notion that policy consists of a number of not very clearly articulated dispositions and is implemented in an evolutionary fashion through a long process of trial-and-error has been termed 'implementation-as-disposition' by Majone and Wildavsky (1979 p. 182).

EXTERNAL CONTROL MODELS

The defining features of external control models are firstly that the overriding determinant of organisational behaviour is for the organisation to survive by reacting to threats from the environment, and secondly that in such circumstances the focus of rationality is at the level of the whole organisation. Such theories fall into three main kinds.

Firstly, Marxist theories assume, a priori, that events inside organisations are a microcosm of events in the wider society. Thus 'internal organisational negotiations and struggles must be seen in terms of extra-organisational positions and resources of the participants – their class membership.' (Salaman 1979 p. 26) Organisations will find it difficult to remain in existence if they fail to assist in the bourgeois control of society. Such radical theories link well with the 'third face of power' posited by Lukes (1974 p. 21 ff); the most insidious and yet most effective use of power is to structure people's perceptions so that they are unable to recognise what is and is not in their objective interests. A second type of external control theory is the resource dependence model (Pfeffer and Salancik 1978) in which a great deal of organisational behviour is treated as a strategy for managing and responding to the various demands made upon the organisation by those agencies upon whom it is dependent for resources. In order to survive, organisations need to be at least minimally effective in meeting these demands or in obtaining resources from elsewhere. Such an approach is also evident in some variations of systems theory, which stress the importance of the environment in which organisations operate. (Katz and Kahn 1978) Thirdly, contingency theories have sought to link particular combinations of features of organisation structure with survival and prosperity in particular kinds of business and environment. (Pugh and Hickson 1976)

Four kinds of example of organisational dependence upon the environment can be found in the literature. Firstly, all organisations are more or less dependent on some other organisations, even if this is only the necesssity to operate within legal constraints, but in the complex public sector which is found in Britain and North America, these dependencies can be multiplied considerably. [7] Kimberly et al (1983 p. 258) have shown how educational service centres in the US have had to walk the tightrope of nurturing relationships with a range of other constituencies at State and local level, all of whose continued support is necessary for survival; moreover the relative importance of these different constituencies can change over time. In Britain, Harrison (1981 p. 9 ff) has shown the extent to which National Health Service employing authorities are dependent upon professional associations for the supply and quality of manpower.

Secondly, and again especially in the public sector, politicians can use the bureaucracy as a scapegoat. Thompson (1981 pp. 277-8) gives the example of the US Congress complaining about the lack of control of the Medicaid scheme whilst simultaneously introducing another virtually uncontrollable health programme.

Thirdly, again in the public sector, regulating agencies come to be dependent upon those whom they are supposed to regulate. Colby and Begley (1983 p. 305) have shown how the operation of certificate of need legislation in the US was based upon the interests of the regulated industry, whilst Richardson and Jordan (1979 p. 113 ff) have shown how (<u>inter alia</u>) the British Ministry of Agriculture is dominated by farming interests.

Finally, consumers are of course part of any organisation's environment, but in the public services it is not uncommon for them to band together in litigation aimed at opposing the implementation of particular policies; Thompson (1981 p. 276) observes that litigation in connection with Medicine and Medicaid programmes siphoned off energy which could have been used to make programmes less costly.

In the context of external control models, 'implementation failures' will be seen to be due either to the fact that non-implementation of a policy does not carry sufficient threat of a loss of resources to the implementing organisation, or that organisational actors have miscalculated the likelihood of such loss, either because they did not perceive the threat as credible or because they had expected to be able to 'free-ride.'(Olson 1965 p. 33 ff) The test of success is therefore whether an organisation implemented a policy well enough to survive and maintain its resources.

THEORIES AND THE CHARACTERISTICS OF HEALTH SERVICES ORGANISATION

A coherent argument can be made that the unitary theories do not adequately describe or predict the operation of health services organisations. It is much more difficult however to argue that any one of the other three kinds of theory described in the preceding sections; adequately serve such purposes, since there is empirical evidence of departures from the unitary model in the direction of all three of the other types of model shown in Figure 5.1. Some of these findings have been mentioned in the preceding sections, but the purpose of this section is to summarise some of the more general characteristics of health care organisations in Britain and North America. This can be done in terms of three kinds of counterfactual to the unitary model, each corresponding to one of the other models.

Firstly, in the direction of pluralistic models there is the fact of internal politics. It is an obvious point that health service organisations tend to be pluralistic even in formal terms, for they consist of a large number of professions, to which loyalty is given more readily than to the organisation (Child 1977 p. 109); the doctrine of

120

clinical autonomy clearly enhances the opportunity
for pluralistic behaviour. In addition to these
formal aspects of pluralism in organisations, a
number of studies in Britain, Canada, and the USA
(Haywood and Alaszewski 1980; Eakin 1984; Saltman
and Young 1981) have highlighted differences of
power and of interests between the occupational
groups in health services.

Secondly, in the direction of bounded rational
models, there is the fact of the limits to human
cognition. Chapters 2, 3, and 4 above have shown
the vague and complex nature of objectives in the
health care field, and it is not surprising
therefore that to date these do not seem to have
exerted a general influence on management behaviour
in either Britain or the USA. (Schulz and Harrison
1983; Schulz, Greenley and Peterson 1983) This
vacuum allows rank-and-file health workers to define
the objectives of health services implicitly.
(Harrison 1981) In addition, health is a powerful
political symbol, (Klein 1983 p. 31) and it should
not be surprising if interested parties are prone to
take symbolic action in this area of policy.

Thirdly, there is the fact of external
politics. The interdependence of complex public
service sectors has already been noted, and this
interdependence is heightened by the role of
external professional licensing bodies, by the need
for referral arrangements between health
institutions, and by the role of third-party payers.
The health field is one where consumer groups have
become particularly active since the late 1960s.

It will be seen therefore that the pluralistic,
bounded rational and external control models are all
capable of throwing some light on the operation of
health services organisations. Indeed, they are not
wholly incompatible. Bounded rational theorists
recognise the importance of internal politics,
(Cyert and March 1963 p. 29 ff) and some models most
notably Crozier's (1964) 'conflictive equilibrium',
stress that although internal politics is a major
explanation of behaviour inside organisations, such
processes are constrained by the need not to call
the organisation's existence into question. There
are normative models of implementation which
recognise the facts of internal politics and the
limitations of techniques. (Stonich 1982)

CONCLUSION: SOME QUESTIONS

It seems possible therefore that the three models, taken together, will help to raise important questions about the implementation of policies ostensibly aimed at improving health services performance. This concluding section raises twelve such questions, the first four of which are prompted mainly by the bounded rational model, the next four by the pluralistic model, and the final four by the external control model. Although the logic of the concept of 'health services performance' is essentially unitary (because it implies that organisations can be straightforwardly assessed in the light of previously-stated organisational objectives), it behoves the critical observer of implementation processes to draw upon whatever theoretical insights are available in examining the activity which occurs under the rubric of 'improving performance'.

1. How has the issue of organisational performance come to be on the organisational agenda?
   Although unitary models suggest that performance is routinely under review, bounded rational models suggest that performance would need to be seen as a problem before any action occurred; social economic or political pressures are amongst the possible explanations for such perceptions.
2. What is the role of information in structuring perceptions about the issue of health service performance?
   At its crudest, there are two opposing ways in which information can be used: either to lead to the conclusion that something is an issue, or conversely, to buttress a conclusion already reached.
3. How far is action taken ostensibly in pursuit of better performance supported by prior analysis?
   Bounded rational models suggest that those confronted with problems are inclined to action before analysis, and that ostensible analysis may well be post facto rationalisation.

4. How far does the action taken ostensibly in pursuit of better performance seem to be primarily symbolic in character?

One answer to the need to respond to a perceived problem is to act symbolically; the creation of new agencies or new posts, changes in formal organisation structure, or the creation of scapegoats are all possible examples of such action.

5. To what extent do different actors favour different concepts of performance?

Pluralistic models suggest that actors will choose and support concepts of 'good performance' which accord with their interests and with their educational and social background. 'If many constituencies have an interest in what a given organisation does, they are likely to use many criteria to make judgements about performance' (Kimberly et al 1983 pp. 251-2).

6. Which actors will benefit as a result of the definition of performance which prevails?

Given that policies concerned with improving performance are almost by definition redistributive, some actors are likely to gain and others lose.

7. What are the types and sources of power employed in order to resolve differences in actors' interests?

Pluralistic models suggest that formal organisational authority may be less important than the resources at the command of particular actors; in addition, the status quo will often provide the opportunity to veto challenges to it, especially where there is a large number of interested actors.

8. What evidence is there of faulty cause/effect reasoning by actors?

There are abundant examples of policies which have either completely perverse consequences or contain perverse incentives. In addition, actions may have undesired side-effects.

9. How far are agencies responsible for improving or monitoring health services performance dependent upon those whose performance they are supposed to oversee?

Monitoring agencies may rely for their

continued existence upon the goodwill of the agencies whom they monitor, especially where the arrangements are voluntary. Moreover, the career prospects of the staf of monitoring agencies may well lie in the mainstream health service organisations.

10. <u>How far are efforts to improve performance in particular organisations limited by dependencies upon outside regulating agencies?</u>
The field of health service organisation tends to be characterised by the involvement of professional associations to whom powers of regulation have been delegated by government, (Peters et al 1978) and which in any event play a part in establishing codes of professional ethics which may be antithitical to some concepts of performance.

11. <u>How far do various actors use indirect health care workers as scapegoats in explaining the need for particular policies ostensivley aimed at improving performance?</u>
The bureaucracy is an easy target in political terms, but other groups not giving direct patient care (such as hospital manual workers) might also be particularly vulnerable to efficiency exercises.

12. <u>Whom do health service organisations treat as their 'client'?</u>
Patients singly, or collectively through consumer and pressure groups, are ostensibly the clients, but it cannot be taken for granted that health care agencies actually behave as if this were, the case, since other external dependencies may be important.

There are obvious areas of overlap between the twelve questions, as between the models, but eclecticism is justified on the grounds that, as Poggi (1965) put it, 'a way of seeing is also a way of not seeing'.

NOTES

1.   It will be noted that the present
discussion concerns a wide range of theories, some
aimed at organisational behaviour in general, others
at more specific processes such as planning or
decision making.   For the purpose of this Chapter,
these differences are not very significant, and the
terms 'objectives', 'plans', and 'policies' are
therefore used interchangeably.

2.   For a characterisation of such rhetoric,
see Fox (1966 pp. 3-4).

3.   The terms 'pluralist' and 'pluralistic'
are often used interchangeably.   In this Chapter,
the former refers specifically to the school of
thought that power is widely distributed, whilst
'pluralistic' is used exclusively as an appellation
for the kinds of model discussion in the fourth
section of the Chapter.

4.   It is perhaps because of this lack of
concern with power that human relations theories are
often seen as unitary.

5.   i.e. 0.99 to the 70th power. This
calculation makes the assumption that actors'
behaviours are completely independent of each
other.

6.   This point illustrates the caveat that
classifying theories has the effect of grouping
together approaches which may have considerable
differences along dimensions not analysed; bounded
rationality theories are often based on stimulus-
response psychology, whereas action theory is
emphatically not!

7.   The State is so deeply involved in
financing and regulating health care in the United
States as not to vitiate this generalisation.

Chapter 6

HEALTH SERVICES PERFORMANCE IN GREAT BRITAIN

Tom Rathwell and Keith Barnard

The creation of the National Health Service (NHS)
in Britain was grounded in an acceptance,
articulated in the National Health Service Act
of 1946, that improvement in the health of the
population was a public responsibility vested in
the government and that access to any public
provision for that purpose should be without any
barrier, but rather according to medical need.
This laudable commitment was unfortunately
accompanied by a misconception: namely that once
health care became a free good, the health of the
people would improve to such an extent that NHS
expenditure would decline because of falling demand
for services.
    Doubts about this soon emerged (Roberts 1952)
and the opposite view, that there would be the
reverse relationship between health services
expenditure and demand, was entertained: the more
resources allocated to health, the greater the
demand for services and hence for more resources.
This seemingly spiral effect of demand upon
expenditure became a cause for political concern.
So much so that in 1953 some five years after the
launch of the NHS, the government established the
Guillebaud Committee to enquire into its cost.
Although the potential of a national health service
to achieve the intentions of the Act remained
unquestioned (the effectiveness of medical care
was assumed) much had already happened since 1948.
The confident initial assumption about its modest
cost when the legislation went through Parliament
was shattered by the need to go back to the
legislature with supplementary estimates during
the first year; the Treasury had decreed that there
would be a ceiling on NHS expenditure; charges
had been introduced either to deter demand (more
crudely, to check assumed abuse of free services),

or to help defray expenditure. Further, a parliamentary committee had questioned whether all possible opportunities were being exploited to secure economies of scale in so large an organisation

By 1953, governments of both persuasions had seen their earnest efforts to control rising costs fail, and the government of the day resorted in Guillebaud to the independent committee of enquiry, whose terms of reference were

> To review the present and prospective cost of the National Health Service; to suggest means, whether by modifications in organisation or otherwise, of ensuring the most effective control and efficient use of such Exchequer funds as may be made available; to advise how, in view of the burdens on the Exchequer, a rising charge upon it can be avoided while providing for the maintenance of an adequate service; and to make recommendations. (Ministry of Health 1956)

When the Committee reported in 1956, it was able to demonstrate that the NHS had a been victim of a profound misperception. Original estimates of cost had been constructed on a very fragile basis from sources of varying quality. There was little solid evidence about consumer behaviour, and until Guillebaud, no-one had tested the explanatory power of inflation rates, as opposed to assumptions about public abuse of a free good or the intrinsic management deficiencies and waste of a public bureaucracy.

The Committee had commissioned a study of health service costs (Abel-Smith and Titmuss 1956), which looked at inflation and demonstrated that between the 1949-1950 and 1953-1954 financial years, the increase in cost at constant prices was only some £11 million, compared with £59 million at current prices. Moreover, as a proportion of gross national product, the cost of the NHS fell from 3.75% to 3.25%, and since there had been a population increase, the per capita expenditure on the NHS at constant prices remained virtually unchanged over the period in question. The Committee was able to conclude that

> the rising cost of the Service in real terms during the years 1948-54 was kept within narrow

bounds, while many of the services provided were substantially expanded and improved during the period. Any charge that there has been widespread extravagence in the National Health Service, whether in respect of the spending of money or the use of manpower, is not borne out by our evidence. (Ministry of Health 1956)

While Guillebaud exonerated the NHS from the more mindless criticisms which had been laid against it, and arguably as a result consolidated it as a national institution (almost a second, secular, established church), it also served to raise a number of issues that were to have continued relevance and visibility. Such issues as the concept of what constituted an 'adequate' service, Roberts' puncturing of the 'Beveridge fallacy' that the NHS would reduce the quanitity of ill-health, how to determine the best use of available resources, whether structural or administrative changes could or would serve the underlying objectives of the NHS, the importance of cost accounting and the tracing of the actual expenditure and the use to which resources were put, central and regional control of expenditure and manpower, and mechanisms for securing better co-ordination and integration of services were never again to be left for long off the public agenda. Guillebaud in retrospect can be seen to have focussed on the importance of management, by proposing a capital programme, planning and the development of control mechanisms. The Committee was sceptical about structural changes, and after reviewing the arguments put forward for change concluded that there was no case to answer. The arguments reviewed by Guillebaud were to surface again over ten years later as the justification for NHS reorganisation.

Thus Guillebaud in a political sense secured the NHS's future. After it, according to Bevan and Spencer (1984 p. 93), 'attempts to constrain spending were replaced by a policy of commitment to real growth; for nearly twenty years from 1957 allocations of revenue increased in real terms by 4% per annum.' Detailed concern for the manner in which these resources were being employed was not initially on the political agenda, but in due course questions began to be raised concerning the efficiency and effectiveness of health services activity and expenditure. (Carter and Peel 1976; Cochrane 1972)

Centrally, ministers did attempt to influence how resources were allocated. The first attempt to direct resources to where they appeared to be most needed was through the capital building programme. 'A Hospital Plan for England and Wales' established as national policy the concentration of medical and surgical specialties on one site, arguing that 'the District General Hospital offers the most practicable method of placing the full range of hospital facilities at the disposal of patients and this consideration far outweighs the disadvantages of longer travel for some patients and their visitors'. (Ministry of Health 1962 p. 6) Thus were professional benefits and social costs built into the decision process.

Whereas the 'Hospital Plan' was function specific in that financial resources were being allocated for a particular purpose within the health service, concern subsequently surfaced over the total procedure for distributing resources because it was seen to perpetuate the advantage of the better resourced areas of the country. The system of allocations built up historically since 1948 was such that those areas of the country which had better initial provision of services got more resources allocated over time without any redistribution in favour of poorer or less well-endowed areas. By the late 1960s this system with its inbuilt distributional bias against the poorer regions was recognised and the 'Crossman Formula' (Crossman 1972) was an attempt to rectify this anomaly. Under the formula resources were allocated to the various regions on the following basis: 50% according to the population served; 25% according to the number of beds; and 25% according to the number of cases treated. It will be noted that this method, whilst an improvement, still favoured the wealthier regions by the weights accorded to beds and cases treated. As long as the beds were there and were used to treat patients, resources provided would sustain the level of activity and hence perpetuate the level of resources allocated. It should also be noted that at the time no one, least of all Ministers, envisaged it as politically and operationally feasible to take resources away. There would only be levelling up between regions over time.

One continuing commonly perceived factor accounting for any shortcomings in the NHS was its trifurcated structure (hospitals, family practitioners, other personal and support services) created by the 1946 NHS Act. Guillebaud's failure to dissipate the concern for structure and expressions of discontent with tripartite arrangements were increasingly heard from the early 1960s. Governmental commitment to change it culminated in proposals for radical alteration in the structure and organisation of the NHS. (DHSS 1972) Their essence was that the hospital based services should be amalgamated with those health-related activities of the local authorities, which left Family Practitioner Services largely left untouched. These changes were effected in 1974.

The rationale for such change was stated to be the desire to integrate and improve the services for patients. Associated with this 'patient-centred' approach was the notion of decentralisation of decision making counterbalanced by greater accountablity 'upwards' that is ultimately to Ministers. It is one thing, however to advocate such a goal, it is another to realise it when no procedure or mechanism previously existed within the NHS for translating goals and commitments into action and change on the ground. Prior to the 1974 reorganisation of the NHS, no explicit operational mechanism existed for achieving 'delegation downwards, accountability upwards' and as its realistion was clearly a 'vital element in the management of the NHS' (Lee and Mills 1982, p. 104), it became incumbent upon the government to find one. One tool which seemed to have particular relevance to the health care field was PPBS (planning, programming, budgetting system), which has been introduced int the 1960s into the US Federal Government, initially in the Department of Defence, where it was seen as having been successful in clarifying objectives and in the allocation of resources, and subsequently in all Departments including Health Education and Welfare. PPBS was regarded as being particularly relevant for the health sector because it encompassed the two main concerns, that is both how policies are developed and the manner in which they are implemented. Thus PPBS was seen to provide 'an appropriate structuring of the planning debate, and to introduce an explicit link between planning and budgetting'. (Lee and Mills 1982, p. 81) In the event, expectations were far greater than achievement; indeed, its acceptance within Health, Education and Welfare was not unequivocal, nor did it achieve the hoped for success. (Rivlin 1977). Disillusionment in the US, however did

130

not prevent other countries from considering PPBS for themselves.

The Department of Health and Social Security (DHSS) in Britain began to experiment with PPBS, or 'the programme budget' as it preferred to call it, during the late 1960s and early 1970s. The DHSS came to the view that programme budgets were inappropriate for operational management and should be used primarily for planning. The rationale for this was that health policies were more usually expressed as services instead of outputs (Banks 1979). Three reasons were put forward for the DHSS using programme budgeting as a planning tool:

1. 'to assist in the DHSS internal planning system;
2. to act as a basis for guidelines to the NHS; and
3. to act as a means for monitoring and control.' (Lee and Mills 1982 p.86)

Thus, increasingly in the 1970s the programme budget became the basis on which guidance on future strategies was issued to the NHS.

The documents prepared on comprehensive statements of Ministers' policies and priorities 'Priorities for Health and Personal Social Services' (DHSS, 1976b) and 'The Way Forward' (DHSS 1977) used programme budgets developed for specific services by the DHSS as 'illustrative indications of the national long-term direction of strategic development'. (DHSS 1977) Here, programme budgeting was considered to be an appropriate mechanism for costing policies, for evaluating priorities within realistic financial constraints, and for examining future strategies. It may also be opined that shifts over time in actual expenditure by health authorities as between programmes (elderly, acute, mental health etc) were the simplest if not the most sensitive indicators of policy priorities being translated into service developments at the local level.

At the same time, as the DHSS became convinced of the merits of programme budgeting, it also addressed the state of planning in the NHS. Health services planning had been hitherto notably fragmented with the dominant mode of planning being hospital or capital planning rather than planning for service development. It was called capital planning primarily because the finance for hospital construction came from capital monies specifically earmarked for building construction. The focus on capital-led planning stemmed from the above mentioned 'Hospital Plan for England and Wales' (Ministry of Health 1962) which articulated the concept of the District General Hospital, comprising an essentialy standard set of medical and surgical specialties serving a designated population and catchment area. Consideration within the document to the health services complementary to those contained within the hospital setting, while present, was muted and indeed overshadowed by the prospect of a national network of major new general hospitals.

This overemphasis on capital planning per se, began to be seen as inappropriate for dealing with the complexities of health service provision. It could be said to reflect an'incremental' approach to planning - a reactive form of planning responding to specific events or crises as they arise - and one that became out of tune with the emerging movement of corporate and public policy planning that evolved out of the 1960s and into the 1970s. The trend was towards a more rational and comprehensive form of planning.

Three interrelated factors can be identified to explain the progression towards, and eventual adoption of, a rational comprehensive planning model for the NHS. Firstly, there was a growing awareness of, and interest in, the ideas associated with corporate management. Secondly, there was increased pressure exerted on all spending departments in central government by both the Treasury and the Public Expenditure Survey Committee to contain costs and to present their financial forecasts in a more comprehensive and rigorous manner. The third pressure for a 'different' planning approach arose because of developments occurring in the NHS. The continued improvement and expansion of medical technology and the costs associated with it, eventually generated some concern for the evaluation of the care being provided and ways of providing care more effectively and efficiently.

Thus the conditions and a rationale for introducing a formal planning system for the NHS were established: acceptance of the need to move away from the fragmented and capital-led planning of the 1960s; the desire to integrate and thereby improve services for patients; and the wish to make the planning of these services more responsive to the 'needs' of the population. This was stated in the following terms: 'health services can only be

evaluated in relation to the identifiable needs of
the community for different kinds of health care
(which) must be expressed in terms of proposed
developments of the components parts'. (DHSS 1972
50-51) In this way planning was seen as a means
through which change could occur whilst ensuring
that the proposed changes were compatible with the
perceived needs of the community. A planning
system was thus complementary to the structural
reform of 1974.

The specific mechanism for translating this
philosophy of planning into practice was described
in the manual 'The NHS Planning System'. (DHSS
1976a) The foundation of the NHS Planning System
was its emphasis upon the 'rational comprehensive'
model of planning. It was 'rational' in that it
assumed that all planning issues could be
objectively appraised and decisions taken on the
merits of proposals. It was 'comprehensive' in
that it implied that all aspects of any particular
issue or topic could be assessed, and the
implication of any course of action weighed
accordingly, thus ensuring that the 'best' or most
appropriate choice emerged.

PLANNING SYSTEMS AND PRIORITY SERVICES

The NHS planning system was seen as an enabling
mechanism, one which would facilitate reshaping
of the services provided and a more effective use of
the scarce resources available for health care. The
introduction of the NHS planning system coincided
with increasing concern in government that the
demand for health services was outstripping the
capacity of the NHS to meet it, and indeed that the
resources available for health care were not
infinite. The response of the DHSS to this dilemma
was the publication of a consultative document,
Priorities for Health and Personal Social Services
(DHSS 1976b) which was based on a series of
programmes or ranges of service for certain groups.
With considerable justification, the DHSS could
claim that this was 'the first time an attempt has
been made to establish rational and systematic
priorities throughout the health and personal social
services.' (DHSS 1976b) The reasons for the DHSS
publishing its strategies for the future in a
consultative document were fourfold: that the
responsibility for developing certain services
rather than others was one to be jointly shared by

the DHSS and the NHS; to indicate the changes in demand, both present and anticipated, of different client groups; to highlight the areas where past neglect had led to deficiencies in provision; and to promote the effective and efficient use of available resources. The cornerstone of the proposals contained in the document was the concept that an appropriate standard of services should be maintained, in the light of known and expected resource constraints.

Together, the documents on priorities and the simultaneous introduction of the NHS Planning System were an attempt by the DHSS to break away from the historically capital-led development of the health service and, in a phrase adopted by Ministers at the time to 'put people before buildings'. It was assumed that, by establishing a standard procedure for health service planning, based upon the twin concepts of rationality and comprehensiveness, services would subsequently be provided according to the 'needs' of the population.

The reaction from within the NHS to the priorities identified was very mixed. Reaction particularly from medical interest groups that were not given high priority led to a modified follow-up publication. 'The Way Forward' (DHSS 1977) - contained a notably more pragmatic approach not only on the question of priorities but also on the issue of standards of service. As Klein (1977) pointed out, '"The Way Forward" is strong on exhortation (but) it is singularly weak on suggestions about how to bring about the hoped for economies'. A basic and fundamental issue thus emerged: the dilemma of imposing a national strategy whilst allowing local discretion. Insistence on a national strategy, for example, could mean that in some places improvements may well be incompatible with local circumstances. Whereas, if the strategy is considered a desirable but non-binding level of service, there is the risk that a continuing debate over priorities will overshadow any meaningful discussion on service improvements.

PLANNING SYSTEMS AND RESOURCES ALLOCATION

Mention was made above of attempts by DHSS to influence the direction or manner in which financial resources were allocated to the NHS. The outcome was the so-called 'Crossman formula' which proved unable to cope with the twin problems of rising

Figure 6.1: RAWP: The Building-up of a Revenue Target

Mid-year estimates of geographic population for each region

Non-psychiatric in-patient services	All day-and-out-patient services	Mental illness in-patient services	Mental handicap in-patient services	Community services (excluding ambulance and FPC services)	Ambulance services	FPC administration services
Population weighted by national usage by each age/sex group	Population weighted by national usage by each age/sex group	Population weighted by national usage by each age/sex group for marrieds and non-marrieds	Population weighted by national usage by each age/sex group	Population weighted by broad cost of national usage by each age group	Crude population	Crude population
Weighted population multiplied by regional SMRs for certain conditions, SFRs for maternity	Weighted population multiplied by overall regional SMRs			Weighted population multiplied by overall regional SMRs	Crude population multiplied by overall regional SMRs	
Population adjusted for inter-regional flow of patients and agency/ETM arrangements	Population adjusted for agency arrangements	Population adjusted for inter-regional flow of patients, agency/ETM arrangements and incidence of 'old long stay' patients	Population adjusted for agency arrangements agency/ETM arrangements and incidence of 'old long stay' patients	Population adjusted for agency arrangements		

Weighted populations combined proportionately to revenue expenditure on each service

If appropriate to region, population adjusted for London Weighting

Revenue available nationally for services distributed in proportion to each region's weighted population

Reproduced by permission of the Controller of Her Majesty's Stationery Office

Key

SMR   Standardised Mortality Ratio
SFR   Standardised Fertility Ratio
ETM   Extra-Territorial Management
FPC   Family Practitioner Committee

demand constantly outstripping the available supply, and the desire for an equitable and efficient distribution of resources according to need. Thus it soon became apparent that a formula which was more sensitive to need and demand was required. Since Crossman had been exclusively concerned with hospital finance, the 1974 Reorganisation also provided an occasion for looking at the issue in whole health service terms.

The response within the DHSS to the pressure for a 'better' method was the creation of a multi-disciplinary, multi-level group, the Resource Allocation Working Party (RAWP) to review the current practice and to assess and recommend an alternative approach. The terms of reference were: 'to review the arrangements for distributing NHS capital and revenue to RHAs, AHAs and Districts respectively with a view to establishing a method of securing, as soon as practicable, a pattern of distribution responsive objectively, equitably, and efficiently to relative need and to make recommendations.' (DHSS 1976c p. 5)

An interim report was presented in 1975 and a final report, was produced a year later; this was of profound importance to the NHS since it advocated the allocation of resources according to a policy based upon 'equality of inputs'. (Lee 1977) The formula developed by RAWP was, as before, essentially population-based and adjusted for differences in age, gender, and marital status. However, the formula went further than that devised by Crossman by introducing a new dimension, namely the weighting of the demographed structure of the population according to the utilization of hospital beds, and the use of standardised mortality ratios as a proxy measure for morbidity. The method is then applied to calculating resource targets for health authorities, derived largely from 'the expenditure it would receive if it were providing services at the national average'. (Bevan and Spencer 1984 p. 100) The manner in which a resource target is developed, is shown in Figure 6.1.

Not surprisingly, the publication of the RAWP Report promoted considerable controversy as its 'Robin Hood policy of robbing the rich to help the poor' (Lee 1977 p. 220) coincided with the beginning of a perceived downturn in health expenditure which meant that health authorities were faced with making decisions on where to cut back, instead of where to spend resources. A detailed discussion and critique of the RAWP Report is beyond the scope of this Chapter (Bevan et al 1980; Lee 1977; Palmer et al 1979; Senn and Shaw 1978; Winyard 1981), but there are a number of salient issues arising out of these various critiques that call for comment and which are directly linked to the overarching question of health service performance in Britain.

The first issue of concern is the deliberate decision not to link the allocation of financial resources with an examination or investigation into how those resources are employed. As the working party stated, 'we have not regarded our remit as being concerned with how the resources are deployed'. (DHSS 1976c p. 8) This was regrettable as the employment of resources must be co-ordinated with their deployment - if one is to determine whether or not these resources are being used effectively and efficiently. One cannot develop criteria for measuring performance without some sort of mechanism for determining whether resources are being appropriately spent. Yet this is precisely what happened, as the RAWP focus was on resource inputs with no attempt being made by the DHSS to transfer the emphasis onto outputs. Thus, as Lee has stated, 'there are grounds for doubting whether a policy of equality in the distribution of 'inputs' would result in an efficient and effective delivery of health services nationwide'. (Lee 1977 p. 221)

The second question is closely related to the first one. This is the non-alignment of the allocation of resources with the NHS planning system, ostensibly the mechanism for determining the manner in which future resources should be deployed. By keeping the two functions separate the seeds were sown for a potential conflict between on the one hand the national desire for 'territorial justice' and on the other hand the local responsibility to develop services according to the 'needs' of the patient. Again, the opportunity to create a direct means for assessing the effectiveness or efficiency of the British NHS was missed.

The resolution of these two major issues presents the DHSS with a basic and fundamental problem: the dilemma of ensuring adherence to a national strategy whilst allowing a considerable degree of local discretion in determining how the strategy should be implemented. The difficulties facing the DHSS can be spelled out in the following manner: insistence on a fairly rigid interpretation of national policy could mean that changes occur in some localities which could be deemed to be inappropriate or incompatible with prevailing local circumstances. However, if national policies seem as desirable but non-binding, there is the danger that they will become meaningless and empty exhortations to health authorities to do better.

THE SEARCH FOR EFFICIENCY

The cornerstone of the reorganisation of the NHS in 1974 was management by consensus in which the NHS was to be managed by a team of equals with no one individual having overall responsibility in the sense that this would apply to a chief executive. Ostensibly the rationale for consensus management was not only to give doctors a greater say in health services administration but also to encourage much better control over the use of central resources. This philosophy was outlined in the 'Grey Book' which stated quite categorically that consensus management is 'essential to the making and effective implementation of decisions for the totality of health care'. (DHSS 1972 p. 15) (For a detailed discussion of team management in the NHS see Schulz and Harrison 1983.)

However by the mid 1970s rumblings of discontent were being heard within the NHS. Briefly, critics were arguing that consensus management, rather than facilitating decision-making, was in fact stifling the procedure. This view was largely the product of a misconception or misunderstanding of what consensus management was all about. For many people associated with the NHS, consensus was an unfamiliar concept. (Royal Commission 1979) Thus was created the myth that management by consensus, in contrast to a hierarchical management arrangement, was unworkable. Paradoxically, Schulz and Harrison (1983) found that according to most management teams, consensus not only worked, but worked well. The response of the Government at that time was to establish a Royal Commission to investigate this and other matters appertaining to the management of the NHS. The report of the Royal Commission on the NHS largely endorsed the critics' views; that the structure of the NHS was in part to blame for its management difficulties. (Royal Commission 1979) The publication of the Report coincided with a change in

government to one committed to bringing, as it was
seen, much- needed efficiency to the public
sector. To this end it initiated a series of
activities within the NHS which were designed to
promote the government's concept of efficiency.
The more notable of these endeavours are discussed
below.

The new government moved quickly to establish
its position by publishing a series of discussion
documents of which 'Patients First' (DHSS 1979)
created the greatest impact. The outcome of this
was a proposal for re-structuring the management
system of the NHS. The main plank of the proposed
changes was that one tier of management should be
abolished and its responsibilities devolved to
District Health Authorities (DHAs). (DHSS 1979)
The proposed changes were ratified in July 1980 and
the timetable for the changeover was fixed for 1st
April 1982. An additional feature of the
restructuring was that DHAs were expected to
delegate most of their powers and responsibilites to
generally hospital-based units of management.

Central to the government view on the NHS was
the 'profound belief that the needs of patients must
be paramount' (DHSS 1979): a re-affirmation of
the philosophy underpinning the 1974 reorganisation. The means for achieving this
objective , in the government's opinion, was to have
the decision-making process as close to the local
community as possible so that the views of those
within the community plus those providing direct
patient care could figure prominently in the
decisions reached.

Concomitant with the decision to change the
structure of the NHS was a concern that planning had
lost its way. It seemed bogged down in a quagmire
of paper with the net result that few if any plans
were ever implemented. And if they were, the
policies or proposals which were implemented seemed
to bear little resemblance to those originally put
forward. In short, planning was thought to have
become too bureaucratic and too inhibiting. (DHSS
1979) Against this background, it was decided
that the NHS planning system would also benefit from
major surgery. The central argument was that the
rational, comprehensive mode of planning was
unworkable and an alternative model which focussed
on the strategic or long-term elements of planning
was proposed instead. (DHSS 1982) This 'new look'
approach to planning became a formal requirement of
the NHS in early 1984. (DHSS 1984)

Consumer participation in the decision-making process in the NHS prior to 1974 was not very strong, and along with the desire to develop health care commensurate with the needs of people it was decided to give the consumer a voice through the medium of Community Health Councils (CHCs). Briefly. CHCs had a responsibility to represent the interests of the public in the health service. There was generally one CHC for each health district and there were reasonably clear criteria established which governed the relationship between these two bodies. (DHSS 1974). Specifically all health authorities were required to consult with CHCs, as well as others, with regard to any policy changes in service delivery. (See Chapter 4 for a discussion on the interrelationships between CHCs and health authorities on major policy issues).

CHCs, as an innovative concept, had problems in establishing their credibility with the NHS. Many NHS administrators viewed the need to consult CHCs on policy issues as an unnecessary and time consuming task and consequently argued that they had outlived their usefulness. (Royal Commission 1979) Even 'Patients First', whilst acknowledging that CHCs had played a useful role, questioned whether there was a need for them now that decision making was to be brought more closely in touch with the needs of the community. (DHSS 1979) Despite these threats to their viability, CHCs are still in existence, as it would appear that the devolution of decision-making down to the local level has not negated the role of the CHC as a representative of the consumer of health care. One could comment that the bringing of the management function closer to the point of delivery of service does not necessarily mean that those who receive or use the services provided are any more likely to be involved in decisions pertaining to those services than hitherto.

Despite these attempts to bolster efficiency in health care management and delivery, the response from within the NHS has again been very mixed. So much so that the government decided that a firmer hand was needed. This firm hand contained a veritable fist-full of initiatives: such as external monitoring through the experiment of a Management Advisory Service, private audit of NHS accounts and Rayner scrutinies; the Regional Review Process; Performance Indicators; and the so-called Griffiths Inquiry. Each of these is briefly discussed, in turn.

'Patients First' suggested that an advisory

group should be established on an experimental basis to monitor 'the quality and efficiency of the ways in which health services are managed and for advising on the development of services at district level'. (DHSS 1979 p. 10) One of these ventures was the Management Advisory Service (MAS), financed by the health authorities to whom it provides advice, whose principle objective was to generate high quality and effective management within a known resource framework. At its roots lay the creation of an information network capable of sustaining the demands of operational managers as well as policy makers. The emphasis was very much on proactive not reactive decision-making. (Mowbray 1983a, 1983b)

The use of private accounting firms to audit the accounts of selected DHAs was another attempt to improve efficiency in health services, through the use of established external agencies. The argument in support of private auditors was that they would be more cost-effective and, not being direct employees of the NHS, they would be less likely to sanction or accept areas of expenditure which did not appear to accord with the authorities' policies.

Rayner Scrutinies were yet another measure to promote efficiency in government, and by implication the NHS. They were called this after the Chairman of Marks and Spencer, who was appointed by the government to apply the business model to the task of improving the efficiency of the government's administrative structure, through the short term secondment of managers away from their normal jobs to make recommendations for economies in specific areas of expenditure. No department of the government was considered to be immune from the attention of tne Rayner team. One area recently investigated in this way was the expenditure by health authorities on advertising for staff. The recommendations arising from this investigation are still to be considered.

In tandem with the introduction of efficiency measures the DHSS sought to strengthen its control of the NHS. This was done in two ways; firstly, there was the creation of an 'Annual Review Process' (ARP) whereby health authorities had to report directly to the DHSS on progress achieved over the ensuing year. The ARP operates on three inter-related levels: the first level is between the Secretary of State for Social Services and his advisers within DHSS and each Regional Health Authority (RHA) chairman and his Regional officers in turn. The next level ARP involves the RHA Chairman, the Regional officers and the Chairman of each DHA and its management team (DMT) within the Region. The final level involves the DHA Chairman, the DMT and the Management Team in charge of each hospital or management unit in the District.

At the first level, RHAs were given specific targets or objectives by the DHSS to achieve over the forthcoming year. These targets or objectives had their roots in national policy and generally reflected DHSS concern over the fact that it appeared that some RHAs were not necessarily placing the same emphasis on these policies as the DHSS. Thus the DHSS was demanding that recalcitrant RHAs make some positive moves towards implementing national policies. RHAs in turn were making similar demands of the DHAs within their orbit, and so on down the line. Failure to achieve previously agreed targets or policies was to be carefully and critically questioned with the onus clearly resting upon the health authorities to show just cause for any shortcomings. How effective the ARP will be in taming recalcitrant health authorities remains to be seen as the first round, in which health authorities were given specific targets and goals, has only recently been completed. The second round to assess their successes and failures has only just begun and it is too early to tell whether or not such a procedure is producing the desired results.

The second mechanism introduced to coincide with the ARP was performance indicators (PIs) which were a set of statistics which would enable local managers to compare their local services with similar areas elsewhere and make judgements on whether or not their services compared favourably with those of their counterparts. The inherent belief in such a system was that supplementing existing management information would enable managers readily to identify those services in need of improvement (see Table 6.1 for a selected list of performance indicators in use). Sceptics have argued however that PIs are essentially spurious measures because they are derived from a suspect data base, reflect hospital usage rather than performance, and bear no relation to health outcomes. (McCarthy 1983; Scrivens and Charlton 1983)

Thus, two conflicting but related concepts are being articulated - one is concerned with the efficient use of resources, the other with the effectiveness of care. They are related in the sense that they share a common interest in the

Health Services Performance in Britain

Table 6.1: Selected Performance Indicators

Acute Hospital Services

Activity indicators (for general medical, general surgery, trauma and orthopaedic, and gynaecology specialties).
1. Urgent, immediate or emergency in-patient admissions in relation to the population served.
2. All in-patient admissions in relation to the population served.
3. Average length of stay.
4. Average number of patients per bed per year.
5. Turnover interval: average length of time a bed lies empty between admissions.
6. Day cases as a percentage of deaths and discharges and day cases.
7. New outpatients in relation to the population served.
8. Ratio of returning out-patients to new out-patients.
9. Admission waiting lists in relation to the population served.
10. Estimated days taken to clear waiting lists at present level of activity.

Financial Indicators (by hospital category)
11. Cost per day and per case by hospital and district.
12. Actual and percentage component costs by hospital.
13. In-patient catering costs per in-patient day by hospital.
14. Domestic and cleaning cost per cubic metre by district.

Manpower Indicators (by District)
15. Percentage breakdown of registered, enrolled, learner, auxiliary nursing and midwifery staff for all acute, and mainly or partly acute hospitals.
16. Ratios of acute sector nursing staff to (i) number of day cases and in-patient cases, and (ii) number of day cases and in-patient days.
17. Ratio of nursing auxiliaries/assistants to domestic staff in acute and mainly or partly acute hospitals.

Services for the Elderly

Financial Indicators
1. Cost per in-patient day by district by

143

hospital.
2. Component costs by hospital (actual and percentage).
3. In-patient catering costs per in-patient day by hospital.
4. Domestic and cleaning costs per cubic metre by district.

Manpower indicators
5. Percentage breakdown of registered, enrolled, learner, and auxiliary nursing staff in geriatric, long-stay and mainly long stay hospitals by district.
6. Ratio of whole-time equivalent geriatric nursing staff to occupied bed days in geriatric, long-stay and mainly long-stay hospitals by hospital and by district.
7. Ratio of returning out-patients to new out-domestic staff in long-stay and mainly long-stay hospitals by district.

Note: These indicators relate only to single specialty geriatric hospitals.

Services for the Mentally Handicapped

Financial indicators

1. Cost per in-patient day by district and by hospital.
2. Component costs by hospital (actual and percentage).
3. In-patient catering costs per in-patient day by hospital.
4. Domestic and cleaning cost per cubic metre by district.

Manpower indicators
5. Percentage breakdown of registered enrolled, learner, and auxiliary nursing staff for mental handicap hospitals.
6. Ratio of whole-time equivalent mental handicap nursing staff to occupied bed days in mental handicap hospital by hospitals and district.
7. Ratio of nursing auxiliaries/assistants to domestic staff in mental handicap hospitals by district.

Note: These indicators relate only to single specialty mental handicap hospitals.

manner in which resources are deployed but they clash because they measure different things. The former is largely concerned with the sort of activity generated per unit of resources (see, for instance, Chapter 3 for a more detailed analysis). The latter focusses on the impact that a particular service has had on the population or sub-group of the population (This issue is discussed more fully in Chapter 2). It has been argued that the PIs developed by the DHSS do not really address either of these issues (McCarthy 1983; Yates 1983) and that they are too narrow in their application (Scrivens and Chartlon 1983).

A number of commentators have argued that the use of PIs should proceed with caution. Their reluctance is based on the following grounds. Firstly, the data upon which they are based are themselves suspect, primarily because they are derived from the Annual Hospital Return (SH3) and the Hospital Activity Analysis (HAA) both of which are notorious for inaccuracies and inconsistencies (Yates 1982), and thus by definition so are PIs. Secondly, they are, unfortunately, institutional based and as such a measure of hospital activity and therefore are not necessarily what they are purported to be - a measure of performance. There are problems of interpretation such that unfulfilled and/or unjustified expectations could result because PIs are concerned very much with the process of health care and not its effect or impact upon people. As Barnes (1984 p. 118) says 'they measure the amount of effort rather than the results of effort'. Finally even PIs have an opportunity cost - a balance needs to be struck between the cost of developing PIs and potentially marginal increases in efficiency in the use of resources. (McCarthy 1983; Yates 1983)

The ledger, however, is not entirely negative as PIs do offer some positive benefits. They can help to focus management efforts especially when confronted with enormous variations in the pattern of care/services available because they help to identify areas for further and more detailed scrutiny. They can help management gather the necessary support for much-needed change or innovation in health care by providing it with credible ammunition to attack those resistant to change. Perhaps their most useful function is that they give management the ability to identify potential problem areas early on. Whilst there is no doubt that PIs are useful it would not do to get them out of perspective for as Downey (1983 p. 119) rightly asserts, 'indicators should not be regarded as absolute measures of efficiency,' since they 'merely provide a preliminary ranking of performance as a basis for further examinations.' PIs are potentially useful management tools and as such are perhaps a prerequisite for an efficient health service. The difficulty with them in their present form is that their potential is largely unfulfilled.

The National Health Service Management Inquiry, (otherwise known as the Griffiths Inquiry after its Chairman) was established by the Secretary of State 'to review current initiatives to improve the efficiency of the health service, and to advise on the management action needed to secure the best value for money and the best possible service to patients'. (Fowler 1983) The Report published in October 1983 (DHSS 1983) contained a variety of recommendations which Barnard and Harrison (1984) have summarised as

Structure and Role Related – the creation of supervisory and management boards within DHSS, the creation of a post of Personnel Director, the specification of responsibilities of chairmen of Health Authories and the creation of the post of General Manager at each level of NHS management including the operational units as designated by DHAs.

The Use of Incentives and Sanctions to induce improved performance.

The Use of a Range of Management Techniques – including quantitative skills such as management accounting, output measurements, meanagement (clinical) budgetting, determination of manning levels, and personnel management such as staff appraisal.

The Greater Involvement of Clinicians in the management process consistent with clinical freedom. (pp. 127-8)

The publication of the Report generated considerable controversy (Rathwell and Barnard 1984; Stewart 1984) but perhaps the most contentious recommendation was the creation of the post of General Manager. (Harrison 1984; Hunter 1984b) As with the other initiatives discussed above it is still too early to comment upon the likely impact of the main recommendation of the Griffiths Report. Informed opinion, however, has asserted that there is much of value in the Report and on that basis it is perhaps best to give it the benefit of the doubt.

EFFICIENCY, EFFECTIVENESS AND EQUITY

Downey (1983) identified three essential questions as being germane to an assessment of efficiency in the NHS: 'first, how adequate is the level of health service provision; second, is it provided economically and efficiently; and third, does it result in the effective delivery of health care?' (p. 118)

It is the last question, he argues, that is paramount to any consideration of efficiency in the NHS, primarily because it also encompasses the other two. The difficulty with Downey's view is that he seems rather confused not only about what the terms efficiency and effectiveness mean but also about the manner in which they are applied. He seems to equate equity with effectiveness, an association which Long (1984) in Chapter 1 refutes. However, as Steele and Dingwell-Fordyce state 'equity as a concept cannot be divorced from consideration of efficiency and effectiveness'. (1983 p. 126) It would therefore seem plausible to argue that considerations of equity should logically encompass the concepts of efficiency, although as Steele and Dingwell-Fordyce (1983) caution 'a fair distribution of resources does not necessarily mean a more efficient or a more effective distribution'. (p. 126).

Any attempt to respond to either or all of these questions concerning efficiency, effectiveness and equity becomes fraught with difficulty. Firstly, there is no apparent consensus on the question of adequacy of the level of provison since to a large extent the totality of care available is directly related to the resources devoted to it and not necessarily to 'need'. There are those who argue that because the resource base is low, the level of provision is low and therefore the solution is to provide more resources. The most recent call in support of increased Government funding for the NHS came from the British Medical Association's 1984 Annual Conference. Secondly, if it is difficult to agree on what should be an adequate level of provision in the NHS, it comes as no surprise that clear differences have emerged on the question of providing that care economically and efficienctly. (Maxwell 1983; Steele and Dingwall-Fordyce 1983)

The ARP and PIs are attempts at getting around the problem but as has been seen they do not appear to address themselves to the central issues, namely, 'that judgements regarding the effectiveness of any organisation involve questions of values and the fact that the values involved are likely to be competing or contradictory.' (Hall and Quinn 1983 p.246) This issue is considered at greater length in Chapter 5. At the end one is left with the seemingly unanswerable question of how does one meaningfully evaluate or assess the performance or effectiveness of the NHS?

IMPLEMENTATION: THE DYSFUNCTIONAL EFFECTS

There have been many different attempts to improve performance in the NHS some of whose objectives have been explicit, others implicit; most however have shown little impact upon events, although for some of the more recent intitiatives it is too early to judge their relative success or failure. This section looks in more detail at just one, on the face of it, relatively simple issue, that of the planning system's ability to shift resources between care groups.

It will be recalled that a raison d'etre of the restructuring of the NHS coupled with the introduction of a rational planning system was the twin desires of integrating and improving the services for patients, as well as making these services more responsive to their 'needs'(DHSS 1980). Given that an integral feature of the NHS planning system was that 'whilst planning needs to be flexible enough to accommodate ... changing patterns of need, it must also be directed towards removing the existing substantial inequalities of care and provision.' (DHSS 1976a p.3) It can be argued therefore that the success the NHS has achieved in implementing its plans is a good proxy for measuring or assessing its performance or effectiveness.

In order to test the assertion that the existence of a formal planning system in the NHS has influenced the delivery of health care provision, an analysis was undertaken of the strategic Plans for RHAs in England. The overriding objective was to record their degree of convergence with and/or divergence from central policies as they currently existed, and to assess whether or not proposals for the future were geared towards a narrowing of the perceived gaps. To do this a profile of current and future revenue expenditure by care/client group was compiled from the available Regional strategic plans. These care/client group expenditure profiles were then converted to show the expenditure per head of relevant population to which the particular service was directed. For example, the relevant population for the elderly was all persons aged 65 and over; for the other categories the total population was used. This conversion was undertaken to enable meaningful comparisons between RHAs. Thus expenditure per head of relevant population allows a reasonable assessment to be made of the extent to which the future programmes of RHAs accord with current central policies and priorities. Equally it should also be possible to draw some tentative conclusions as to whether or not RHAs were deploying the resources available to them in an efficient and effective manner in the sense of reaching out to those most in 'need'.

An initial comparison between Table 6.2, showing the base line expenditure for those RHAs for which data was available, and Table 6.3 indicating the projected expenditure per RHA by care/client group, suggests that most RHAs have accepted the argument put forward in support of central priorities in health care and therefore are planning to channel resources into these programme areas. Table 6.4 sets out a slightly different way of interpreting the proposed changes in expenditure over the planning period. It shows the percentage net change in the proportion of expenditure between that currently allocated to a specific care/client group and the projected expenditure. These different methods of analysis would suggest that RHAs do appear to heed central policies. To draw such a conclusion, however, would be premature. It is misleading in that, although a comparison between Tables 6.2 and 6.3 shows an overall increase in expenditure per client group, the increase may be due to a declining population base, rather than to any apparent desire on the part of RHAs to conform to central policies. Even Table 6.4 which presents a much rosier picture must be viewed with caution.

To illustrate these points further, the analysis below focusses on general and acute hospital services, and services for the elderly and the mentally handicapped, the intention being to indicate whether or not significant shifts have occured or are programmed to occur in the pattern of resource distribution for priority groups in the

TABLE 6.2: Current Expenditure per Head by
Programme (1976/77), £ Sterling

Service Region	General and Acute	Elderly	Mentally Handicapped
Northern	38.4	61.3	3.9
N E Thames	58.7	71.3	4.1
S E Thames	54.9	72.4	4.1
S W Thames	40.2	58.8	8.3
Mersey	45.5	66.4	4.3
N Western	44.2	50.6	3.8
Yorkshire	40.6	61.7	3.5
Trent	33.8	60.1	4.0
West Midlands	48.7*	63.2	4.1
Wessex	32.5	63.0	3.5

Source; Regional Strategic Plans

TABLE 6.3: Projected Expenditure per Head by
Programme (1988), £ Sterling

Service Region	General and Acute	Elderly	Mentally Handicapped
Northern	48.0	79.3	5.1
N E Thames	59.9	111.9	5.3
S E Thames	58.2	86.1	5.3
S W Thames	41.4	69.1	8.1
Mersey	41.1	84.9	5.4
N Western	57.7	73.7	4.5
Yorkshire	47.0	76.4	4.7
Trent	45.6	79.7	5.7
West Midlands	57.7*	87.3	5.0
Wessex	36.1	81.7	4.3

The Strategic Plans for Oxford, East Anglian, South
Western, and North West Thames RHAs were prepared in
such a manner that extracting the necessary
comparative data was not possible.
* Includes maternity

Health Services Performance in Britain

TABLE 6.4: Percentage Net Change in the Proportion
of Expenditure per Client Group 1977-1988

Service Region	General and Acute	Elderly	Mentally Handicapped
Northern	-0.5	0.9	0.2
N E Thames	-4.7	3.3	0.7
S E Thames	-1.5	1.4	0.8
S W Thames	0.9	0.2	-0.3
Mersey	-2.7*	1.5	0.2
N Western	-0.3	1.2	-0.4
Yorkshire	-2.3	0.8	0.4
Trent	-0.2	0.8	0.3
West Midlands	-2.2*	2.2	0.1
Wessex	-5.3	2.9	-1.0

The Strategic Plans for Oxford, East Anglian, South
Western, and North West Thames RHAs were prepared in
such a manner that extracting the necessary
comparative data was not possible.

* Includes Maternity
Source: Regional Strategic Plans

NHS.
     Comparison of the Tables indicates, without
exception, an increase in spending per head of
relevant population for general and acute hospital
services. Whilst the magnitude of the projected
increase in expenditure varies between RHAs, it is
salutory to note that even those RHAs considered to
have an excess of acute hospital services (generally
regarded to be the four Thames Regions, (DHSS 1976b;
London Health Planning Consortium 1979)) have
planned an increase in spending. This does appear
to run counter to the counsel of earlier central
guidance for 'rationalisation and pursuit of economy
in the acute sector.' (DHSS, 1977, p. 13) It could
also indicate that the desire for efficiency may
well be overridden by other and possibly more
powerful forces. This theme will be addressed more
fully later in the Chapter.
     The elderly and younger physically disabled is
the only care group for which a significant increase
in expenditure is forecast for most RHAs over the
planning period (see Table 6.3). This increase in
expenditure fully accords with central priorities;
indeed it would appear that the elderly is one
priority in which the centre and the RHAs can agree.
However, this picture is to some extent an
illusion. In the Thames RHAs, for instance, the
projected increase in expenditure is due more to a
forecast decline in the elderly population than any
attempt at re-distributing resources. Nevertheless,
increased priority for the elderly is shared by both
the centre and the RHAs; partly a consequence of the
expected increase in the elderly population –some
4.5% by 1991 (Craig 1983) and the very effective
lobbying of certain pressure groups such as Age
Concern, and other concerned organisations and/or
individuals. (The Health Services 1983)
     The planned-for increase in expenditures for
mental handicap is the least of all the priority
groups, and because of the anticipated decline in
population some projected increases are, in reality,
reductions in cash expenditure. In other words, the
actual projected increase in expenditure is so small
that if the forecast decline in the population does
not occur, some RHAs would be spending less per unit
of population on services for the mentally
handicapped, than they do at present. The evidence
suggests that the NHS does not necessarily place the
same priority on this service as does the centre.
     It was argued earlier that by investigating
whether or not the delivery of health care was

meeting the 'needs' of the population (equity) one was also directly addressing issues of efficiency and effectiveness. It is clear from the foregoing analysis that these questions are not very high on the agenda. There are some tangible factors which appear to explain this lack of progress towards effectiveness in health care. There are also a number of intangible factors which impinge upon outcomes. These are now considered in some detail.

EFFECTIVENESS: AN ELUSIVE GOAL!

Despite the evidence that more resources will be made available for the priority groups, this analysis indicates that little change in the distribution of expenditure in favour of these groups will be forthcoming in the foreseeable future. The apparent failure in shifting proportionally more resources into these policy areas is partly due to a lack of enthusiasm for central goals at the local level and partly due to a failure to appreciate the importance played by the less tangible elements of power, prestige, and professionalism in inhibiting genuine attempts at reform. (Rathwell 1981) Thus the creation and implementation of a planning system, such as that operative in the NHS will not, of itself, produce the desired · result. Hyman (1982) has identified five factors which he argues can undermine the validity of planning. These five factors may be briefly summarised as: inappropriate data; conflicting objectives and alternatives; technical complexities; weak theoretical base; and quantitative simplicity. These inhibitors will now be discussed in more detail, as all of them, to a greater or lesser degree, can be argued to be responsible for the general lack of confidence expressed in the NHS planning system, and in its failure to effect an overall shift in priority areas towards the needs of care/client groups and for a more efficient use of the available resources.

The first of the debilitating factors identified is inappropriate data. Data are not something that the NHS lacks; in fact it can be argued that it has a surfeit of data but little information. The major problem is that the data routinely available in the NHS are often considered to be inappropriate for use in planning and management. They are inappropriate because the data collection process was designed to provide information for central requirements, not for local planning and management purposes. A Regional Administrator had this to say on data collection in the NHS; it 'represented the aggregate over time of unsystematic requests for information on aspects of health services activity covering – but far from comprehensively – both patient and staff activity. Fortuitous accretion was the hallmark of a process determined from the top downwards, on the basis of national requests and priorities, but with no regard to the needs of the operation level, who provided the data.' (Fairey 1983 p. 181) This state of affairs was evident at the time that the NHS planning system was introduced, as the following comment from the Regional Chairman's Inquiry in to the working of the DHSS in relation to Regional Health Authorities published in 1976, makes clear; 'we (got) a strong impression that much information is demanded quite unnecessarily – either from a mistaken sense of need, or as a continuing legacy of one ad hoc request.' (quoted in Fairey 1983 p. 181)

Given this background, it is not surprising that many of the plans produced were not implemented. If the database on which the planning problems are analysed and assessed is inadequate, then it is reasonable to assume that any measures put forward in response to the problems will themselves be suspect. Lack of confidence in the data inevitably leads to lack of confidence in the published product of any planning system employing such data. It is encouraging to note that the question of a fragmented information base is currently under review (Körner and Mason, 1983), but past performance suggests that argument over the legitimacy of the base data has undermined many a plan to reform it. This leaves open the thorny but necessary question of whether or not the NHS would use the new data. Furthermore, it is precisely this issue which is thwarting attempts to develop a set of performance indicators which would be generally acceptable to the NHS.

The second factor is concerned with conflicting objectives and alternatives; the specification of objectives and the generation of options is one of the major requirements of planning. It is also one of the most problematic and conceptually difficult requirements to fulfil. Three reasons can be offered in support of this argument. Firstly, until recently, policy makers in the NHS have traditionally thought in terms of service inputs – the components necessary to provide

a particular service - but are now being asked to
think in terms of the impact of the services they
are providing. For many policy makers such
shifts in conceptual thinking have proved to be
particularly difficult to achieve, even where the
database to support such a change is available.
Secondly, the involvement of different groups in the
planning process has meant that a number of
conflicting perspectives of the problem to hand are
proffered. This raises questions of not only what is
the problem, and what are its contributing factors,
but also leads to different views on the objectives
to be achieved, and the alternatives available for
their realisation. Doctors, for example, will
generally look at an issue from a clinical or micro
perspective - is it in the best interests of the
patient? Health administrators in contrast tend to
take a macro view - does it conform with existing
facilities and services and can it be afforded?
Such differences in perception are not easily
overcome, as each side is usually determined that
their interpretation of the issue is the most
appropriate. In short, there are not only
professional differences to accommodate, but also
differences of scale.

The third factor is the inherent cautiousness
or conservatism of most decision makers. They wish
to be remembered for their achievements, not their
failures and therefore will be cautious about
setting objectives that are unlikely to be achieved.
What is at stake is their credibility as managers.
For this reason most policy makers are 'inclined to
support traditionally popular and successful
programmes and promote their extension into areas of
need, or favour minimal adaptations to make such
programmes more efficient and effective rather than
risk new or unproved approaches to health problems.'
(Hyman 1982 p.153) This has obvious implications
for planning. Indeed, it would not be uncharitable
to suggest that this cautiousness and conservatism
towards priority decision making was largely
responsible for the lack of movement by RHAs towards
improving those priority groups identified by the
DHSS. Achievements may be measured more in terms of
organisational harmony and stability and not by
degree of radical change made.

The third confounder is technical complexity;
planning requires a continual commitment from both
decision makers and planners. Unfortunately, there
are a number of barriers which affect the required
close working relationships of the two. Firstly,

they are working towards different time horizons. The decision maker, on the one hand, under pressure from patients and/or providers of care, wishes a quick resolution of the problem. The planner, on the other hand, is reluctant to put forward any alternative until satisfied that the problem has been fully analysed and the possible implications of any alternative properly assessed. Thus the desire for a quick but effective solution conflicts with the time horizon required for a considered assessment of the problem.

Another area of potential difficulty between the policy maker and the planner is one of perspective; they tend to conceptualise problems quite differently. Take, for example, the specialty of general surgery in an average District General Hospital, which shows the following characteristics: long waiting lists, high rates of bed occupancy, pressure on nursing staff, and so on. The clinician in charge or the nurse manager may see the problem as one of the shortage of beds, lack of sufficient nursing staff, lack of adequate resources, or all three: an essentially simplistic view of the problem. The planner would tend to regard the views of the clinician or nurse manager as being solutions to an unknown problem. Thus, the planner would argue that the symptoms of the problem require extensive investigation before one can state categorically what the problem is, and what remedies might be most appropriate.

Finally, there are the analytical and technical complexities of planning itself: in particular the absorption of systems ideas and the use of computers or mathematical computations. A key component of planning is the use of modelling, and either analogue or symbolic models are used in an attempt to mirror the real world. The systems model is key, according to Bailey, because it 'is the interface between the real world for all its ramifying complexity, and our simplified schematized investigations of it.' (Bailey 1975 p.8) Bailey in his supportive comment on systems modelling has (inadvertently) highlighted a critical reason why modelling often fails to provide the solution. The failure stems from the fact that they are essentially 'simplified schematized investigations' of complex issues. In other words, in order for the model to replicate or simulate the real world, a series of often questionable assumptions must be made. The consequence is that because the model was considered, rightly or wrongly, to be based on unrealistic assumptions, little credence was placed on the result.

The fourth confounding factor is the weak theoretical base; according to Hyman (1982) 'most analysts are skilled in model building'. Whilst this statement may be true for personnel employed in the NHS as operational researchers, it certainly is not true for the majority of its planners. (Rathwell 1984) McNaught (1981) puts forward the proposition that the lack of 'expertise' amongst NHS planners is a consequence of a 'generalist cult' among administrators who are capable of a variety of tasks and activities, but not necessarily expert in any. Because 'policies are settled by bargaining between groups, with their own interests and frames of reference, rather than by analysis' (Brown 1975 p.233) it is not surprising that it has proved very difficult in the NHS to develop more sophisticated and specialised approaches to health planning.

When the NHS planning system was introduced, emphasis was placed upon the inter-disciplinary nature of the activity, whilst acknowledging that members of planning teams were to be chosen for their 'professional skills and knowledge of the Service, not for technical planning expertise.' (DHSS 1976b) The necessary technical expertise was to be supplied by specialists in information handling and planning, a commodity which was, and still is, in very short supply in the NHS.

It has been suggested that the emphasis on the interdisciplinary characteristic of planning has been misplaced because the evidence suggests that such teams do not operate in a 'rational' manner. (Glennerster 1983) Observers of the multi-disciplinary approach to planning in the NHS postulate that it was the dominance of one particular profession (medicine) which mainly dictated the plans and policies put forward. (Glennerster 1983; Haywood and Alaszewski 1980; Illsley 1980; Rathwell 1984) As Lee and Mills (1982) have observed, 'despite the existence of the NHS planning system and provision for the systematic consideration of projects, planners had difficulty combating the ability of influencial clinicians to bypass the planning system and lobby decision makers directly.' (p.141)

The last intervening variable is quantitative simplicity: planning requires quantitative measures that are comparable. Unfortunately comparable measures are difficult to obtain, and indeed quantification may not be possible. This difficulty in providing suitable and appropriate quantifiable measures has led critics to question the validity of planning. 'Current solution techniques, particularly mathematical programming, are limited to a small subset of the total spectrum of problems to which the process of systems analysis or rational planning might be applied, and in most cases operate under such restrictive assumptions and over simplifications as to make the solution obtained only of general relevance to the problem.' (Hemmens and Lathrop quoted in Hyman 1982 p.154)

Both 'Priorities for Health and Personal Social Services' and 'The Way Forward' in an attempt to facilitate comparison between priority client groups placed a great deal of importance on centrally derived norms or standards as the basis for their programme budgets. The trouble with relying on norms as a de facto basis for comparison is that it is presumed that norms or standards have their roots in practical experience and that the variable concerned is an accurate proxy for all the factors which determine workload. Additionally, there is the real danger that by translating an average into a norm or standard, one moves (illogically) from the position that something is the case to the statement that something ought to be the case. (Harrison and Rathwell 1980) When this happens, particularly for norms for which the underlying assumptions have not been made explicit, it tends to undermine their credibility for normative use. This is of particular importance in the NHS as strategic planning has tended to be dominated by an over-reliance on norms as the main basis for determining a desirable level of service. Glennerster (1983) in examining the strategic plans of one particular RHA found them to be almost entirely based on central planning norms, so much so that the plans 'turned out to be very crude rationing devices poorly reflective of the centre's priorites (and) unresponsive to local situations that were far too complex to work out at Regional level.' (Glennerster 1983 p. 83) The arguments apply with equal force to the more recent attempts to develop the performance indicators since they are essentially similar in derivation.

CONCLUSION

It would be reasonable to conclude that the application of rational planning to the NHS has not been an unequivocal success. The attempt by the DHSS to introduce the twin concepts of 'rationality' and 'comprehensiveness' into what was previously a very fragmented approach to planning has at best only been partially fruitful, in as much as it has at least brought to the forefront the debate over which services/facilities deserve priority status. (Glennerster 1983) However, there has not been the hoped for accord between those priorities determined centrally and those perceived to be important locally. The available evidence, in the form of the examination of RHA strategic plans suggests that differences over which service should be given priority vary widely not only between the centre and the periphery, but also between RHAs.

Five reasons have been propounded for the apparent failure and these have been found to have some substance when applied to the NHS. The convoluted database of the NHS, developed and sustained by incrementalism is not conducive to a systems orientated approach to decision making. Secondly, planners have not been given very clear organisational objectives within which to plan. Thirdly, most of those involved in planning in the NHS have either not understood the analytical and technical complexities of systems planning, or have not been able to convince their colleagues of the merits of such an approach. Fourthly, the planning process has often been undermined by the ability of one professional group or another to circumvent the system and ensure that its views are given precedence. Lastly, there has been an over-reliance upon norms or standards, many of dubious origins, as the basis for analysis and comparison of appropriate levels of service.

It could be argued that for most of the initiatives on efficiency and effectiveness described herein, the jury is still out in the sense that on the one hand the evidence which suggests that the measures are not what they purport to be is largely circumstantial. On the other hand, there is sufficient interest in them to give them the benefit of the doubt and to try to implement them. In any case it would be premature to either condemn them out of hand or to endorse them uncritically.

It has been postulated that health services performance entails more than just a concern for efficiency and effectiveness and that it should also include considerations of equity. If one accepts this, there then arises the question of how to implement such a policy. There can be no definitive procedure for effecting this philosophy primarily because decisions on equity, efficiency and effectiveness take place within a political environment, and against a background of continuing changing values and perceptions.

Nevertheless it is possible to offer for consideration a 'performance checklist' (Table 6.5) which seeks to provide a framework for judging the provision of health care services. The checklist has four components: firstly a theme which espouses a particular philosophy of providing services that provide value for money and meet the needs of the public, whilst ensuring that no one is unduly disadvantaged as a result of the spatial distribution of such services.

The second component is couched in the form of two challenges for health authorities: rationalisation and collaboration. Health authorities can no longer look foward to 'new' monies to finance improvements in health care. The current economic climate is such that they face a declining resource base rather than an increasing one and so any desire to make improvements which have financial implications means that the additional monies required must be offset by savings elsewhere. For most DHAs this implies that rationalisation of services can never be completely removed from the agenda. The second challenge, collaboration, refers to the fact that health care cannot be divorced from the wider milieu in which it is placed. Lalonde's health field concept (1974) and Long's diamond model (1984) admirably demonstrate this wider association. Therefore any attempts to improve the efficiency and effectiveness of health services must take cognizence of the fact that in many ways the outside enviroment is just as crucial to the hoped for outcome as is a purely health-related initiative. Failure to recognise this has been obvious implications, especially for questions of effectiveness and, to a lesser extent, efficiency, when the outcome of a measure of service is dependent outside factors. Thus cooperative arrangements between the health sector and those organisations which have complementary responsibilities, such as local authority social services departments, is essential.

The third item on the checklist introduces some criteria for evaluating the acceptability of health policies, whether local or national in outlook. Social acceptability implies that the policies under

Table 6.5: A Performance Checklist

1. THEME
    Efficiency and effectiveness founded on the
    concept of equity in health care.

2. CHALLENGES FOR HEALTH AUTHORITIES
    - Rationalisation of services
    - Inter-organisation collaboration

3. CRITERIA FOR POLICIES
    - Socially and politically acceptable
    - Technically sound with professional
      commitment
    - At a realistic and affordable cost.

4. QUESTIONS TO JUDGE THE RELATIVE MERITS OF
    PROPOSALS
    - Who will benefit and who will not?
    - In what ways and to what extent?
    - How many will benefit?
    - At what cost?

consideration are in tune with local or community
needs; whereas political acceptability means that
no one group is likely to be unduly disadvantaged
vis a vis any other. It also suggests that the
changes being proposed have been thoroughly
discussed with all those who have an interest in the
application of such policies so that the necessary
steps can be taken to defuse as far as possible any
opposition. It is possible to minimise opposition
by demonstrating that the proposal(s) are
technically sound; that is capable of being
introduced within the existing infastucture and
available technical limitations. Demonstrating this
is very important because without this step it is
most unlikely that one would be able to carry the
professional staff crucial to the implementation of
any policy.
    Having considered the viability of policies on
the grounds of social and political acceptability,
technical merits and professional involvement, the
final hurdle to overcome is the question of cost.
Some programmes may be very costly but are
determined to be socially and politically
acceptable, to fall within known technical limits
and to have the backing of the professions
involved. It may prove to be very difficult to rule

out such a proposal on the grounds of cost alone. While costs are clearly important, they should not be the determinant of the viability of policies, especially if the concept of equity is acknowledged to be a governing factor in health services provision.

The final section of the checklist highlights a number of questions with which to judge the relative merits of proposals. The list is by no means exhaustive, and there may be other questions one would wish to include, but Table 6.5 represents a useful starting point. Consideration of who benefits and who does not, from any proposal, are important at any time, but take on greater meaning in times of economic constraint where the outcome is often seen in terms of 'winners' and 'losers'. It is equally necessary to identify who 'wins' and 'loses' and what the likely impact of the proposed changes will be for each group, in order to be able to demonstrate that the implications of the proposal have been thoroughly thought through. It is argued that cost should be considered last because it should not be seen as the over-riding factor which determines whether or not a programme goes ahead.

While greater efficiency and effectiveness in health services is to be welcomed such objectives should not overshadow or distort the basis or philosophy for providing such care. In the case of the NHS its performance should not be judged on questions of efficiency and effectiveness alone but rather the emphasis should be directed more towards the broader question of equity.

Chapter 7

HEALTH SERVICES IN CANADA

Geoffrey Mercer

It has been widely claimed that, in comparison with
the polar extremes represented by the 'free
enterprise' system in the United States and the
'state controlled' health service in the United
Kingdom, Canadian health care has devised its own
middle ground. (Horne 1980; Weller 1980; Crichton
1984; Vayda and Deber 1984) Moreover, it has been
suggested that the organisational distinctiveness of
the Canadian system is matched by an enviable
performance on a range of key health status and cost
criteria. (Canada: Health and Welfare 1974; Evans
1982a) In this Chapter, some of the central
features of the growth and current organisation of
the health services in Canada are highlighted. As
in Britain and USA, the 'politics of performance
evaluation' have proven contentious and problematic.
Two difficulties stand out: firstly, how to balance
central and local powers and responsibilities; and
secondly, how to reconcile 'public accountability
and professional autonomy'. (Klein 1982 p. 388) The
striving for an improved performance across this
North Atlantic triangle has to be set both within
the similarities in post-1945 social development as
well as against the specific economic, political and
social circumstances of each society. The
discussion of health service performance in this
Chapter therefore attempts to draw attention to
those aspects which mark off, in a comparative
sense, the Canadian system from its counterparts in
the USA and Britain.

OUTLINE OF HEALTH SERVICE ORGANISATION

The validity of the claim that a distinctive
approach has been adopted in Canada rests squarely

in what Horne (1980) describes as the 'joint venture' that has emerged between the public, private and voluntary sectors. At the popular level it is associated with the establishment of health insurance (Medicare) on a countrywide basis, with 'medically necessary services' provided 'free' at the point of delivery. 'In essence, the public sector assumes major responsibility for financing the costs of health services, while the private (for-profit) and voluntary (non-profit) sectors together assume major responsibility for the production and delivery of health services.' (p. 197) This public sector takeover of health insurance during the 1950s and 1960s significantly altered the mix of public and private involvement in health funding and regulation. By the late 1970s, three quarters of total health spending was accounted for by the federal, provincial, territorial and local governments. (Canada: Health and Welfare 1983a p. 26) The federal proportion of this total health bill between 1971 and 1981 has fluctuated between 41.0% and 46.4%. Over the whole post-war period the general trend has been for health costs to become a more prominent item in both the federal and provincial budgets. At the national level, such expenditure as a percentage of Gross National Product has risen from 2.9% in 1950, to 5.6% in 1960, through to 7.5% in 1980, and to a provisional figure of 8.4% in 1982. (Canada: Health and Welfare 1983a; Evans 1982a Table 1) At the provincial level in 1980, the health cost element in the gross domestic product varied from 5.3% in Alberta, to 13.9% in Prince Edward Island. (Canada: Health and Welfare 1983a p. 46) On average almost one quarter of all provincial government spending is on health.

The greater part of the federal expenditure on this sector is derived from general taxation, while the provinces generate their revenue from a wider array of sources, including sales and income taxes, and in the case of British Columbia, Alberta and Ontario, from health premiums. Over the past fifteen years, political concern has been growing apace with the increase in health funding. At the same time, both opinion polls and national investigations report solid, general support for the Canadian health care system. (Canada: Health and Welfare 1980; House of Commons 1981)

The private element in health care is represented by the one quarter share of total health expenditure, and more obviously, by self-employed,

Health Services in Canada

fee-for-service physicians. Each of the ten provincial plans provides a fee schedule which lists the insured procedures as well as the appropriate payment. Medical practitioners bill the provincial plan, not the patient. There are several exceptions to this pattern. Around 10% of physicians do not participate in, or 'opt out' of their provincial plan. A further variation is the practice of 'extra-billing', where a physicians seeks direct payment from the patient of an amount over that prescribed in the fee schedule of the insurance plan. The scale of extra-billing varies considerably across the country, but even in those provinces where it is more prevalent, such as Alberta and Ontario, the proportion of total services affected is probably less than 5%. (Canada: House of Commons 1984) The permutations on the relationship between provincial plan, patient and physician are numerous; extra-billing is restricted to a handful in Quebec because patients cannot claim reimbursement from their insurance, while in Alberta, Saskatchewan, New Brunswick, Nova Scotia and Prince Edward Island, it has been permissible for medical pratitioners to remain in the plan and extra bill.

A further practice that has attracted much federal government criticism is the imposition of 'user charges' on patients. A number of provinces have employed these on the grounds that they raised necessary revenue, or that they inhibited unnecessary utilisation of hospital and medical services.

The method of remunerating physicians, as well as the possible growth of direct charges on patients, have helped to keep health policies in the political spotlight. The power of the medical lobby in health policy making is as well established in Canada as elsewhere. (Grove 1969; Charles 1976; Tuohy 1976; Taylor 1960, Coburn et al 1983) So too is the pre-eminence of the 'medical model' of health. (Blishen 1964; Clute 1963; Coburn et al 1981) In consequence, the intersection of the public and private sectors in Canada produces a confrontation over the costs and control of health care. 'Sole source public funding and public fiscal responsibility coexist uneasily with decentralised and essentially private authority over patterns and levels of service delivery - a coexistence in which friction is inevitable and occasional conflict unavoidable'. (Evans 1982b p. 178)

The voluntary sector plays a lesser role,

although its influence is widely spread, and in
particular fields can achieve a marked impact. It
is visible through the activities of voluntary
organisations such as the Canadian Red Cross
Society, the Canadian Heart Foundation, and the
Victorian Order of Nurses. In addition, there is a
noteworthy voluntary presence in hospital
administration. In 1974, 8.1% of hospitals were
privately run (for profit), 7.2% were federally
owned and administered, with the remaining 84.7%
classified as public hospitals recognised by the
provincial authority. In terms of the proportion of
hospital beds, the public sector dominance is even
more complete. However, these public hospitals are
largely operated by non-profit organisations (for
example, religious, lay, municipal and provincial),
although dependent on public sector funding.

If the joint venture depends on a distinctive
division between the public and the private sectors,
it is also broadly constrained by the often
difficult and disputed constitutional relationship
between the federal and the provincial governments.
The British North America Act of 1867 provided for a
variant of federalism in which the provincial
responsibility for health services was countered by
the dominance of the federal government's revenue
raising and spending powers. (Stevenson 1977) With
health matters regarded as of little significance to
the federal government, but rather a local, or
private concern, the provincial responsibility in
this area was established. (Aucoin 1974; LeClair
1975) More recently, this has meant that the
federal government exerts strong influence over
health policies, because of the power of the purse,
although the constitutional jurisdiction lies with
the provinces. Hence federal accountability for the
performance of the health services is still lacking.
In consequence, policies for the health services
have increasingly been a bone of contention between
a federal authority intent on 'nation building', and
the growing expression of 'province building'
ambitions outside Ottawa. These have been spurred
since the 1960s by such developments as the
resurgence of separatist feeling in Quebec, and
rapid economic growth in several western provinces,
such as Alberta with its oil wealth.

Over the period since the end of the Second
World War, there have been significant changes in
the organisation of Canadian health services. A
system which in the 1930s was quite close to that of
the United States took off in a fresh direction.

The provision of health care on a wider and more equitable basis was regarded as central to post-war policy making. In the words of the Canada Health Act 1984, 'the primary objective of Canadian health care policy is to protect, promote, and restore the physical and mental well-being of residents of Canada and to facilitate reasonable access to health services without financial or other barriers.' (Section 3) Public discussion of health care in the 1940s and 1950s bore full witness to its important role as a vehicle in promoting both social stability and national unity. It was to be a major element in post 1945 social reconstruction. (Tsalikis 1982a) As in Britain and the USA, the expansion of the health services in Canada came under attack from the late 60s onwards. The changing fortunes of the economy, and its downturn in the 1970s, provided the justification for policies at both the federal and provincial government levels designed to cut back on the growth of social welfare expenditure in general. Closer inspection of developments in the period after the Second World War highlights both the trend towards the 'provincialisation', as well as the 'politicisation' of health care. (Weller 1980) Questions about the link between the funding and control of the health services become politically more acute. Indeed, several commentators see the Canadian health services at a cross road. (Evans 1982a; Vayda and Deber 1984) Is the joint venture still delivering the goods? How can the system be made more efficient? Is the 'medical-industrial complex' out of control?

HEALTH SERVICE EXPANSION: THE ROAD TO MEDICARE

Before the Second World War government involvement in the organisation and development of health services was limited mainly to public health regulations. (Tsalikis 1982a; LeClair 1975) A federal sortie into health benefits in 1935 was repulsed by the Supreme Court as ultra vires, and although there were innovative plans for health insurance in some provinces, these were never implemented. A combination of opposition from important vested interests (mainly insurance companies, but with some medical support) plus the uncertain financial capability of provinces to undertake such a scheme blocked any progress. (Torrance 1981; LeClair 1975) Tsalikis (1982b) argues that the necessary cooperation between the

167

levels of government only emerged as the pressures on existing health services grew in the inter-war years. He lists, 'epidemics and severe health problems among the destitute; the inability of remote and economically unattractive communities to secure continuing medical services; the need of industrialists with remote or risky operations to secure medical services and thus attract labour; and, finally, the increasing difficulty of hospitals to secure funds for expensive medical technology'. (Tsalikis 1982b pp. 127-28) Since the existing mixture of public and private schemes to help with health cover appeared unable to provide the funds required by hospitals, or the level of remuneration thought reasonable by physicians, let alone an adequate level of health care for ordinary Canadians, the pressure to find alternative policies built up.

The special conditions created by the Second World War provided a further boost. In addition to the stimulus to re-think intergovernmental relations, there was considerable federal interest in the possibility of formulating a range of social welfare measures as part of a post-war reconstruction of Canadian society. (Crichton 1976; Tsalikis 1982a; Aucoin 1974) The prospects for the development of a countrywide health service initially seemed favourable, with evident public support expressed in opinion polls for a system of health insurance. The proposals were to founder on concerted opposition from the provinces on constitutional and funding grounds, and the unease of the medical profession over this 'unknown octopus' in the health field. Private capital appeared divided over the issue, and although organised labour was supportive, it did not impress itself on the debates. (Tsalikis 1982a; Walters 1982; Taylor 1978)

In the wake of its failure, the federal government took another course to sponsor the growth of the health services. In 1948 a system of health grants was agreed. These took the form of ad hoc payments, and those concerned with hospital construction and professional training support became very potent factors in stimulating the expansion of the health sector. They began a trend for the funding of provincial health services on a conditional or cost-shared basis. The monies were largely used to strengthen the position of specialised, hospital based, curative medicine. Scientific medical research and education was also given a boost through other programmes where the federal government had scope for independent action. (Aucoin 1974)

The vast federal potential for health funding proved equally crucial to the establishment of: firstly, hospital insurance as laid down in the Hospital Insurance and Diagnostic Services Act 1957 (HIDSA); and secondly, full Medicare, which became operational in 1968 after the passage of the Medical Care Act two years earlier. Nevertheless, the strength of the provincial opposition to federal interference had been sufficient to greatly delay the implementation of 'approved' health insurance schemes across all of the provinces. Indeed it was the case with both hospital and medical insurance that the federal government only acted after various provinces had experimented with their own schemes. The innovative policies of the Cooperative Commonwealth Federation/New Democratic Party (CCF/NDP) government in Saskatchewan exerted a particular impact. (Taylor 1978) However, the involvement of the federal government through an extensive financial commitment to share costs, provided that provincial plans satisfied certain conditions and, ensured that there was a measure of uniformity in the schemes implemented across the country.

HIDSA and the Medical Care Act therefore extended both federal funding and regulation of the health system. The cost-sharing arrangements introduced with Medicare meant that the federal government met half of the costs generated in the provincial plans. Herein lies the much referenced notion of the 'fifty cent health dollar', since every dollar of health care costs incurred in the insurance plans was to be matched by the federal exchequer. In addition, the sharing formula negotiated between governments included a 'Robin Hood' element designed to redistribute monies from the richer to the poorer provinces – especially those in the Atlantic region. The federal government saw this as an opportunity to play a special role in promoting national unity. (Weller and Manga 1983) Its contribution to each province's costs under the 1957 Act was calculated on the basis of the 'national and provincial per capita costs of insured services multiplied by the number of insured persons in each province'; while under the 1966 Act the basis was 'the national per capita cost of insured persons multiplied by the number of insured persons in each province'. (Aucoin 1974 p. 61) The change in calculating the formula between 1957 and

1966 indicated that the attempt to promote inter-provincial equity had not achieved the level of redistribution intended. (Weller and Manga 1983)

The federal share of health costs in both pieces of legislation was conditional on what have come to be called the 'principles' of Medicare. Although contained in the 1957 Act, these were not spelled out in detail until 1966. They are: comprehensive coverage for medically necessary services, which is related to the notion that there will be no financial barriers to impede reasonable access; universality, or at least 95% enrolment on uniform terms; portability of benefits across Canada; and public, non-profit administration of the plan. (LeClair 1975) The definitions have left scope for various interpretations, especially on whether user charges inhibit access to services, and these disputes provided the immediate justification for the 1984 Canada Health Act.

The impact of the hospital and health insurance programmes was felt across a number of areas. Positive evaluations concentrated on the considerable increase in funding of the provincial health care systems. This encouraged an expansion in the number of facilities and personnel. More investment in hospital and medical services was equated with an increase in equity and effectiveness. In those terms, progress was being made. The bed-per-population figure rose steadily between 1950 and 1970, especially among the acute care services. And indices of hospital utilisation grew steadily through the 1950s and 60s. (LeClair 1975 pp. 42-48; Soderstrom 1978 chapter 2) Since the control of costs was not a prime objective in health policy making, but rather the search for equity, the generally positive evaluation was understandable.

Yet a contrary interpretation was developing. Concern for greater efficiency in the allocation of resources to health was linked with inter-governmental conflict. An important feature of both the HIDSA and the Medical Care legislation was that it provided for the growth of some services and completely ignored others. Expansion of the 'general' and 'allied special' hospitals was cost-shared, but tuberculosis and mental health hospitals, along with nursing homes and institutions for the aged were not recognised as hospitals under the terms of the 1957 Act. There was little incentive to control 'shared' expenditure, and no encouragement to develop 'non-shared' services, even though these might be cheaper or more effective alternatives. While Medicare extended insurance cover from hospitals to physicians' services, it still omitted proven beneficial services, such as nursing homes, and skilled health practitioners, such as nurses. The last of the provinces to join the Medicare scheme did so in 1970, but by then the Canadian economy was becoming less buoyant, and there was mounting criticism that public expenditure was a burden that must be reduced. The attack on 'unproductive' state intervention was a theme that won political adherents across most liberal democratic societies. In Canada, references to the 'health costs crisis' came to dominate both federal and provincial government thinking. The post-war phase of expansion in the health services gave way to a period of containment.

MEDICARE: COUNTING THE COSTS AND CREDITS

The figures in Table 7.1 illustrate the growth in health care expenditure in recent decades. Although the data for the period prior to 1960 refer only to personal health spending, the general trend of increasing costs is demonstrated. The rate of growth accelerated on two occasions: first, in the 1950s, and second, in the late 1960s. There is further possibility that an upward surge has taken place in the early 80s. Equally notable however, is the picture of health costs in the 1970s. While the total bill continued to rise, health expenditure as a percentage of GNP held steady. The rise in health spending in the late 60s sparked off a stream of reports, inquiries and white papers which constitute a barometer of official concern, as well as the focus for a changing approach to the growth and organisation of the health services.

A clear indication of the search for alternative solutions was provided in the several reports and recommendations of the Task Force on the Cost of Health Services which was set up in 1968 on the initiative of both federal and provincial governments. Their Report (Canada: Health and Welfare 1970) included considerable criticism of the lack of cost-conscious planning, and detailed many ways in which managerial efficiency in the health services might be promoted and improved. They focussed on the need for: a change in funding arrangments, both to contain costs in general, as well as to reallocate resources away from the

Table 7.1: Health Care Expenditure in Canada, 1950-82

Year	Total ($ Millions)	Per Capita ($)	% of GNP	% GNP in USA
Personal Health Expenditures				
1950	535.4	39.0	2.9	4.5
1953	734.9	49.5	2.9	4.3
1956	988.2	61.5	3.2	4.6
1959	1362.5	77.9	3.9	5.3
All Health Care Expenditures				
1962	2561.4	137.6	6.0	5.6
1965	3415.0	173.5	6.2	6.2
1968	4909.7	236.9	6.8	6.8
1971	7122.3	329.9	7.5	7.7
1974	10247.5	457.6	7.0	8.1
1977	15532.6	666.8	7.4	8.8
1980	22178.6	921.4	7.5	9.5
1982*	30087.7	1220.2	8.4	10.5

* provisional figure

Sources: 1) National Health Expenditures in Canada 1970-1982 (Canada: Health and Welfare 1983a) for Canadian data 1960-82, and for US data 1970-82.
2) Evans (1982a)

NB: official statistics issued by both the Canadian and American governments have been subject to continuous revision

acute hospital sector; manpower planning, especially to improve labour productivity and flexibility; regionalisation of services, including the growth of community health centres; and public participation to enhance the legitimacy of the containment proposals.

Criticism of the lack of efficiency and accountability in the use of health expenditure was increasingly linked to the questionable effectiveness of some of the high-cost services. The Lalonde Report, 'A New Perspective on the Health of Canadians' (Canada, Health and Welfare 1974) attracted considerable interest because of its

forceful promotion of the 'health field concepts',
and the suggestion that a law of diminishing returns
applied to the funding of curative, hospital based
facilities. Further improvements in health status
must be sought in changing people's (unhealthy)
lifestyle, and in reducing the risks arising in the
physical and social environment. In terms of the
present discussion, the Lalonde Report is noteworthy
for its attempts to offer criteria by which to
evaluate the successful provision of services.
'There are three overall indicators of the level of
health services: the ratio of various health
professions to the total population, the ratio of
treatment facilities to the population, and the
extent of pre-paid coverage.' (p. 26). The Report
goes on to compare the Canadian experience with that
of Australia, Denmark, Sweden, the UK and the USA.
'In hospital and medical insurance coverage, Canada
equals the best of the five countries chosen for
comparison; it leads in respect of physicians, is in
the middle rank in respect of hospital beds, and is
second only to Australia in nurses. Since the
countries chosen are among those with the best
health care services in the world, there is no doubt
that, by the four measures used ... Canada is among
the world leaders.' (p. 27) The cost-efficiency of
the Canadian health system is not made the subject
of international comparison. Instead, after
reporting the per capita cost of health care for an
individual Canadian, and a family of four, the
judgement is offered that, '(t)his is a substantial
sum by any measure.' (p. 27)

If the evaluation of health service performance
rests on such general criteria, it is perhaps
because Lalonde had a more pressing intention: to
check health 'cost escalation'. (Evans 1982c) From
this perspective the current problem for governments
is to enhance cost control through managerial
efficiency. The Lalonde Report is notable therefore
not merely for the expression which it gives to a
multi-factoral approach to health, but for the
manner in which it encapsulates a gathering view
that closer control of health care funding was
imperative, and that this should be allied with
renewed efforts in health planning, such as
regionalisation of health authorities, an integrated
informationm system, and manpower planning. (pp. 28-
9)

On another level, the 'New Perspective'
indicated the growing opinion of the federal
authorities that they should disengage more from the

current funding arrangements, and must be situated
within the protracted and acrimonious
intergovernmental negotiations then in progress to
find an alternative to cost-sharing. The new
formula finally agreed was set down in the Federal-
Provincial Fiscal Arrangements and Established
Programmes Financing Act 1977 (EPF). It is widely
argued that EPF represented a new stage in health
policy making because of the far greater
possibilities that were provided for meaningful
provincial control and financial responsibility for
their health care systems. (Weller and Manga 1983;
Vayda and Deber 1984)
     EPF represented a more direct approach to
stemming the flow of federal monies to the
provinces. It sought also to place the transfer on
a more predictable basis, as well as one which set
limits any increase in the federal contribution.
In addition an attempt was made to 'promote cost-
cutting and greater efficiency by instituting a
system where any savings would accrue to the
province, and by eliminating the distortion of
provincial spending that had resulted from the
distinction between insured and non-insured
programs, such as home care and extended health
care, that had been a part of the shared-cost
programs'. (Weller and Manga 1983 p. 233) The Act
also provided for more equitable transfers between
the provinces.
     As befits a measure negotiated primarily by
finance ministers rather than their health
colleagues EPF is extremely complex. It replaced
previous cost-sharing arrangements with a cash
transfer and Ottawa relinquished substantial 'tax
room' - in other words, the provinces were provided
with sources of tax revenue previously collected by
the federal government. 'The cash payments
consisted of "basic cash" contributions,
"transitional adjustments", and "levelling"
payments.' (p. 233) The cash transfer was related
to previous funding levels, plus an allowance for
the rate of growth in GNP. Other arrangements were
designed so that no province lost revenue under the
new scheme.
     The implementation of this 'block funding'
rather than 'cost-sharing' formula has been
generally accepted by the provinces as a welcome
recognition of their constitutional responsibility
for health. What did not subside was the provincial
complaint that the level of federal funding, and its
rate of increase, were both too low. Charges and

countercharges have filled the air about exactly how much of health expenditure is now provided out of the federal exchequer. Much depends on whether the surrendered tax room is taken into account. The general trend appears however to have been for an initial increase in the federal contribution, and for a subsequent decline to pre-1977 levels. (Canada: House of Commons 1984). The provinces have been further angered because federal spending is geared to the rise in general prices, whereas health cost inflation has always been much higher. Any expansion in the health services must then be met increasingly from provincial resources.

Not that the federal government was satisfied with the impact of the new funding arrangements. Its charge that the provinces were misappropriating transfer monies intended for health into other fields was not supported by a review of selected aspects of the health services conducted by Justice Hall. (Canada: Department of Health and Welfare 1980) The Liberal Government continued to claim that it was picking up too high a proportion of the health care budget, and in 1982 it amended the financial formula built into the 1977 EPF Act. The provinces were incensed by this unilaterial action which, by tying federal contributions more closely to the overall growth of the Canadian economy, probably ensured a much increased provincial burden over the ensuing five years. (Weller and Manga 1983; Canada: House of Commons 1984)

The supposition that the federal government would adopt a lower profile on health matters did not occur. There had been periodic complaints through the 1970s that the underlying principles of Medicare were being watered down, or negated, by the practices of extra billing, user charges and health premiums. These came to a head in 1983 when Alberta's health minister announced the first across-the-board system of hospital user fees. He presented this policy as a response to the underfunding of the health care system that had followed the federal government's reduced financial support, and as an attempt to induce a greater degree of cost consciousness among consumers of health services. The Federal Minister of Health responded with a position paper, 'Preserving Universal Medicare'. (Canada: Health and Welfare 1983b) She (Mme Begin) argued that user charges and extra billing were threatening the underlying principles of Medicare, and that fresh legislative action was required to preserve its social effectiveness. This led to the introduction of the Canada Health Act which became law in 1984. Despite the grand title, its ambitions were largely restricted to the funding arrangements between federal and provincial governments. Since it had no legal authority to ban any of the offending health charges, it followed a previous course, and made federal funding conditional on meeting the Medicare principles. For those provinces which continued with extra billing and user charges, the extimated cost of these activities would be withheld unless and until the provincial government took corrective action. In July 1984 the first monthly penalties totalling $9.5 million were announced. Ontario, British Columbia and Alberta alone stood to lose $8 million. While some provinces have changed course there is little indication so far that richer provinces such as Alberta and Ontario have been persuaded to bow to federal pressure.

The point was raised earlier in the discussion that the climate which gave form to Medicare altered at the moment of its implementation. What had been acceptable in terms of health service expansion, was then re-interpreted as an economic liability. Nevertheless, general support for Medicare has endured, although the success and acceptability of its implementation has been the subject of some dispute. That the basic principles offer the proper criteria for evaluating the organisational performance of the health sector was central to the Canada Health Act. Not that the definitions of the original four principles - to which 'reasonable remuneration' for physicians has been added (Canada: Health and Welfare 1980 chapter 3) -are without ambiguities.

Lest the criticism swamp the achievements, hospital and medical insurance gained widespread acceptance because care was made available to all residents of Canada, and without an excessive financial cost to the patient. Similarly the standards of hospital care and administration were improved. A detailed monitoring of provincial conformity with Medicare aims was not however possible because of the lack of information. There always has been variation across the provinces but all were supposed to stay true to the basic conditions.

The principle of universality, or unimpeded access to services has been a central issue in the dispute over user charges and extra billing. A number of studies have been conducted into the impact of user charges, and these have generally concluded that they reduce access disproportionately among the less well-off. (Barer et al 1979, 1982; Badgley and Smith 1979; Canada: Health and Welfare 1980) Although there is no accurate information on the extent of extra-billing, it does appear to be concentrated in some areas, and in some specialisms. Evidence on the situation in Ontario where the yearly extra-billing income was estimated at $50 million, suggested that slightly less than 15% of physicians in the province as a whole were involved but that in the City of Toronto this included 91% of anaesthetists and 71% of gynaecologists in Metropolitan Toronto. (Canada: House of Commons 1984)

Another source of dissatisfaction has been the uneven distribution of physicians and medical facilities. Many of the northern and more rural regions of the country are not well provided with physicians, although there is a highly favourable ratio of physicians-to-population in the country as a whole. In 1982 the ratio was 1 : 522. (CMA 1984b) Under Medicare, several of the worse-off provinces recruited many new physicians; Newfoundland reduced its population per active physician from 1,991 to 708 between 1961 and 1978, New Brunswick improved from 1,314 to 890, while a better-off province such as British Columbia reduced its ratio over the same period from 758 to 528. (Canada 1964, Canada Health and Welfare 1980)

The comprehensiveness of health care was defined by the Royal Commission as 'all health services, preventive, diagnostic, curative and rehabilitative, that modern medical and other sciences can provide.' (Canada 1964 p. 11) In the Medical Care Act, the phrase 'medically necessary services' was employed and the interpretation left largely to medical opinion. This has been regarded by many commentators as a lost opportunity to turn the Canadian health services away from medical dominance, and towards less costly alternative methods of care.

When Justice Hall conducted his review in 1979 and 1980 of the health services, he received many submissions on the problems arising out of the portability provisions in Medicare. These were mainly administrative, for example, 'uninsured transients from Ontario (where there is a system of health premiums) seeking care in Prince Edward Island; ... students at out-of-province universities; or ... patients who did not have the insurance identity card with them.' (Canada: Health and Welfare 1980 p. 39) In such cases, the patients might well find themselves with a demand for an advance payment. This is a problem which has created 'great annoyance with many Canadians.' (p. 40)

Justice Hall gave short shift to the idea that the public administration (non-profit) of the provincial insurance plans might be beneficially transferred to the private sector, as recommended by a number of insurance and medical bodies. He noted that the average level of administrative costs in the ten provincial plans was 2.5%. This was significantly lower than that achieved by the pre-1958 insurers in Canada, or currently in the USA where non-profit and commercial insurers reported administration costs of 7 and 18% respectively. (pp. 43-44)

The disputed 'fifth principle' suggested by comments in the Medical Care Act was 'reasonable compensation' for physicians. In his 'commitment for renewal' of the health services Justice Hall treated adequate medical remuneration as central to the survival of Medicare. There is evidence that physicians' earnings have moved unevenly. (Evans 1982a) These had been rising in the 1960s, but Medicare appeared to provide a further stimulus, so that physicians did better than most other groups in Canada. But from the 1970s onwards, physicians' net incomes rose more slowly than the consumer price index. This relative decline seemed justifaction enough to the Canadian Medical Association (CMA) that doctors were not being 'adequately compensated'. The CMA further argued that fee-schedule settlements imposed on physicians provoked strikes and other forms of 'job action', opting out and extra billing, and migration between provinces or abroad - to the USA in particular. (CMA 1981 1984a) Hall's Report (Canada: Health and Welfare 1980) refused to speculate on how the remuneration of physicians might be calculated except to recommend that 'the Provinces should develop a mechanism to ensure reasonable compensation'. (p. 29) Since neither of the parties to the dispute have been willing to accept compulsory and binding arbitration, the problem remains.

The question mark that hangs over Medicare's implementation and accountability very much depends on the interpretation of, and attachement to, these principles. Although Medicare's principles are

couched in the language of social equity, its
implementation has been increasingly bound by
pressures to increase efficiency, and reduce its
costs to governments.

TOWARDS MANAGERIAL EFFICIENCY?

In this section, discussion will concentrate on
provincial initiatives to improve the performance of
their health care systems. With no two provinces
pursuing exactly the same path, illustrations of
health policies span examples of interesting
practice - without attempting to provide a detailed
picture of any single provincial system. The
developments selected for mention here fall within
three broad areas: the organisation and delivery of
services; financial management; and manpower
planning. 'Rational' models of health planning have
increasingly provided the framework within which
these issues are considered.
        The time was ripe for provincial stock-taking.
Talk of 'spiralling health care costs' was very much
in the minds of governments. Inquiries mounted in
Ontario, Quebec, Manitoba, and British Columbia were
indicative of the concern. (Ontario 1970; Quebec
1970; Manitoba 1972; British Columbia 1973).
Extracts from the White Paper on Health Policy
issued by the Government of Manitoba are
illustrative of wider provincial thinking. Health
planning was proferred as a rational strategy for
allocating resources in an efficient as well as
equitable manner. It was further advanced as a
mechanism that would enhance the accountability for
health service organisation and delivery by bringing
government, health providers and consumers into the
process.
        The White Paper hammered home the message that
health costs were escalating in directions where
effectiveness was questionable. Moreover, the
distribution of services, which is so important in
Canada - the second largest land mass in the world,
yet with a population of only 25 millions - was
criticised for not ensuring equitable access, and
for reflecting the health needs of the population.
Fresh policy directions had to be attempted that
would both control costs and improve access to
health services.

        The heart of the matter is that the system has
    largely lost touch with any method of a simple

and effective kind for providing incentives to use scarce resources efficiently. The system is fragmented where is should be unified.... The consequence is that in many of its separated parts the system lacks a mechanism for choosing the less expensive rather than the more expensive way of doing something equally well. It is uneconomical - drastically so. (Manitoba 1972 p. 2)

The White Paper's planned reforms included both an extension of ad hoc measures to contain costs and particular services as well as a more fundamental re-organisation which would regionalise and integrate the provision of care via 'district health systems'. These districts were to be run by community boards representing both users and providers of health services. They would be provided with a global budget for current and capital expenditure, and it would be their decision how to allocate that money. In a similar vein, the White Paper argued for more community health centres as a way of holding down costs while increasing accessibility. (p. 45)

ORGANISATION AND DELIVERY OF SERVICES

Manitoba's record of successful implementation of policies for a more integrated health care system was not impressive, even under a sympathetic NDP government. (Black, Cooper and Landry 1978) By 1977, when a Conservative administration came to power, only three health districts had been established in the province. The major urban area, Winnipeg, stood apart and most initiatives embraced rural areas. A similar experience with Community Health Centres restricted their number to nine, and several of these did not properly qualify because of the small number of physicians and nurses attached to them. Throughout these years, such innovative attempts to bring about structural change were starved of resources, and plagued by problems whereby integration was advanced through 'administrative fiat' rather than a clear understanding of its basic objectives, or how to promote them, as with the intended link-up between public health and social services. (Ryant 1977) There was also a familiar tale of physician opposition. Problems in achieving an acceptable balance between local and central control and accountability applied as forcefully within provinces, as between the provincial governments and their federal counterpart.

If, in Manitoba, the translation of health planning theory into practice was very limited, a comparison with Quebec's experience is instructive because of the manner in which it enthusiastically implemented planning techniques. A highly interventionist government took control in the 1960s, and set about producing a comprehensive programme for health care. This followed recommendations from the Commission of Inquiry on Health and Social Services, the Castonguay-Nepveu Report. (Quebec 1970) When Castonguay entered provincial politics and was immediately appointed Minister with responsibilities for health the prospects for change seemed excellent. The guiding concern for health care was that it should be provided in a comprehensive package linking health and social services; that it be decentralised in its management; that it provide for meaningful consumer participation in defining priorities and allocating resources, as well as in evaluating their efficiency and effectiveness. This heralded a design for comprehensive decentralisation. (Gosselin 1984)

A new Ministry of Social Affairs was created with a strong planning function. The Health and Social Services Act, 1971 sought to reorganise its services along three main lines. Firstly, the local community service centre (CLSC) was to act as the screening agency for the more specialised services. It was 'designed to be the backbone of the primary health care system, linking preventive and curative services and providing continual patient care....The CLSC stressed the team approach'. (Tsalikis 1982b p. 151) At a second level were 32 Departments of Community Health (DSC), which were under the wing of acute care hospitals, and had responsibilities for preparing, implementing and evaluating appropriate health programmes in their area. On a further level were 12 Regional Councils for Health and Social Services (CRSSS) with an overall consulting and co-ordinating role. (Godbout 1981)

In a review of the regionalisation experience in Quebec, Gosselin (1984) documents some of the ways in which consumers and health care providers were involved in the planning of the health services. In his estimation this has been most successfully achieved at the 'primary level of health care and social services' although 'opposite conditions prevailed and still exist at the

secondary- and teriary-care levels. Patients' needs
continue to be defined in the organisations' own
terms and the services to be offered from the
organisations' own perspectives.' (p. 22) So far
the experience of decentralisation has not confirmed
the original expectations.

Even so, Gosselin's assessment is relatively
more optimistic than that offered on consumer
participation in CLSCs. Godbout talks about a
unique institution being 'quickly marginalised in
the health care network.' (1981 p. 153) By 1980,
about one half of the 210 CLSCs that the government
had planned for were in operation. Their
distinctiveness lay in the majority representation
of citizens and users on the boards of directors, as
well as in the emphasis on 'la medicine globale'.
Such organisations are always likely to provoke a
counter-move from physicians, and the establishment
of private 'polyclinics' - with a group practice
offering a full range of traditional and family
medicine - proved so successful that these now
outnumber CLSCs by 4 to 1. (Tsalikis 1982b pp.
151-52) Less than 2% of all general practitioners
work in CLSCs. Yet out of 172 CHCs in Canada as a
whole, serving some three and a half million
people, one hundred were in Quebec. (pp. 153-4)

There are also claims that consumer
representation has been difficult to translate into
consumer power to bring about notable change in the
administration of hospitals. Godbout (1981)
highlights the 'consolidation of bureaucratic and
professional control', while Eakin's research
pointed to a 'deterioration in the administrators'
sense of organisational control, a weakening of the
boards' authority over physicians, and a
concentration of decision-making outside of the
boardroom.' (1984 p. 221) Rather than mobilise
local interests, user representatives were more
often co-opted into the organisational view of
health problems.

Regionalisation experiments in other provinces
seem equally patchy. In British Columbia, the idea
is said to be on the agenda again, although without
definite policy proposals. (UBC 1982 pp. 59-61)
Ontario has set up 26 district health councils in
the past decade. These have an advisory capacity,
and in recent discussions on the future direction of
that province's health services provided information
on the needs of their district. While they have
acted as an occasional buffer between the provincial
health ministry and the local population, and are

regularly consulted on developments in services, their executive power is negligible, and their future role in any further decentralisation uncertain. (Ontario 1983)

Ontario's pluralistic approach in the provision of health services is illustrated in a recent commitment to community health centres and health service organisations (HSO). Exactly how many resources will be devoted to such primary care initiatives is at present uncertain. In 1984, there were 18 HSOs (capitation funded) and 11 CHCs (programme-based budget), but these covered no more than 200,000 people, and their future seemed dependent on resources being transferred from other areas. Only one was sponsored by a physician, with the rest promoted by community groups. In addition, there is a crucial barrier to the growth of capitation funded organisations because in Canada the basic fee-for-service principle in provincial health insurance plans allows little scope, or incentive, to pass on savings and thereby attract more patients/members. At the same time, the Ontario Ministry of Health envisages that CHCs are most appropriate for groups with poor health status, or who otherwise are low users of health services. (Ontario 1983, 1984b) Both HSOs and CHCs are expected to provide medical and nursing care, together with social service contributions on, for example, nutrition and family guidance. In general, attempts to move away from the 'medical model' of health and illness have been less ambitious in Ontario than comparable schemes in Quebec.

The experience of regionalisation and community health centres in these provinces has been less encouraging. In Manitoba, the experiments never really took off, while in Quebec the progress has been uneven, and the support of the provincial government not always enthusiastic. With professional opposition, some association in the public mind with 'services for the poor', and no detailed confirmation of their superior efficiency and effectiveness to other forms of service provision, the community health centres face an uphill struggle to become more generally established. In similar fashion, the introduction of decentralisation into the health decision making process during the 1970s has yet to justify its advance billing in anything like full measure. Some aspects of regionalisation have been confounded by new information and control systems, which make for at least as significant central direction, and undermine the emphasis on consumer and provider participation at the service levels. 'There is also a distinct possibility that the search for greater equity in resource allocation between and within decentralisated units might tend to diminish flexibility for meeting local needs.' (Gosselin 1984 p. 8)

Regionalisation of services and the development of alternative forms of care were of course central themes in the Lalonde Report. But what of the implementation of health promotion, and how far has the environmental and lifestyle emphasis been demonstrated, if at all? The 'appeal of programmes emphasising self-responsibility and lifestyle modification during times of restraint' (Love et al 1984 p. 304) has been widely remarked upon. Not that this commitment has led to any noticeable reallocation of resources to health promotion programmes. (Evans 1982c p. 328)

The still generally favourable public support for health promotion was reported in a series of health study conferences held in Ontario in 1983, and in the countrywide debates leading up to the Canada Health Act 1984. (Ontario 1983; Canada: House of Commons 1984) An amendment in terms reminiscent of the Lalonde Report was incorporated in the Act's statement of health care objectives. The federal government has also promoted campaigns against smoking and alcoholism, and has tried to persuade Canadians to improve their general physical fitness. At the provincial level, it has failed to convince all governments to introduce seat belt legislation. In Ontario, Ministers of Health were still talking in 1983 of establishing 'health promotion and disease prevention as a major priority'. (Ontario 1983) In 1984 a new group was set up within that Ministry charged with the implementation and co-ordination of plans in this field. The five key areas to be addressed were: improved physical fitness; anti-smoking; alcohol abuse, better nutrition; and increased awareness about individuals' responsibility for their own health. These represent a partial take-up of the main recommendations from the provincial study conferences. The focus has been directed primarily for health education campaigns rather than intervention at the level of the wider social environment. Although the Ontario Minister of Health indicated that health promotion would be one of his first priorities in office, there has been as yet no significant financial commitment.

Implementation of the Lalonde Report's suggestions was always problematic, with health care a provincial rather than federal responsibility, and with several possible 'readings' of its policy implications. Those interpretations hostile to the overly medical orientation of health services and to their impact on health costs have been sidelined. Evans (1982c) has argued that health care providers have simply added a range of new preventive medicine techniques to their armoury. The prospect that the future benefits of preventive and health promotion activities will more than compensate for current increases in expenditure is less than convincing (p. 344)

The Ontario experience appears to be fairly typical. The 'New Perspective' has provided ample scope for governments to be seen to be doing things that few would denigrate, and which cost very little. Their symbolic impact is indicated by the failure to seriously dent the proportion of resources devoted to the traditional hospital and medical services. Their effectiveness remains unproven.

Analysis of the 'failure' to implement these reforms in the delivery and organisation of services, or of the problems in achieving the anticipated improvements, cannot be separated from their associated costs and efficiency. Selected aspects of the financial management of the health services are now examined.

FINANCIAL MANAGEMENT

The management of health care systems has in the past decade gradually become wedded to the application of strategic planning techniques, albeit in varying degrees. The Ontario government has bemoaned the orientation to crisis management in the health sector. With gathering problems, it has enthusiastically embraced the precepts of long range planning. (Ontario 1983) Studies of British Columbia report a similar shift in recent years with the proclaimed intention of making health management more rational. (UBC 1982) Changes in organisational structures, co-ordinating mechanisms and information systems were introduced in line with the new emphasis on financial management and more particularly with the 'supply side dynamics of rationing and control'. (p. 33) 'Cost control managers' have displaced predominantly medically qualified administrators in health ministries. The performance climate projected by the BC Ministry of Health has therefore been firmly tied to fiscal restraint in order to make the most efficient and effective use of existing resources. (UBC 1982 p. 59)

The two largest items in the provincial health budget are for institutional care (especially hospitals), and professional services (especially physicians). Since the introduction of Medicare these two categories have accounted for more than one half of all health expenditure. The predominant management approach has been 'top down'. 'The successful public control mechanisms have been global limitations in the form of restraints on institutional operating budgets or new capital acquisitions, attempts to reduce numbers of health manpower, and tight negotiation of fee schedules'. (Evans 1982b p. 179) There have been few attempts to closely monitor or evaluate the efficacy of different health services, although government publications now place more weight on explicit performance measures.

The provincial funding responsibility over hospitals starts with the negotiation of an operating budget. Capital expenditure is calculated quite separately. As a rule, the operating budget is determined at the beginning of each year, but it has been regular practice for these to be adjusted either during, or at the end of the year, if the hospital finds itself in difficulty. The scale and rate of increase in hospital budgets, together with their apparent resistance to prudent management, has encouraged repeated efforts to place hospital budgetting on a more rational basis.

The initial allocation of funds has long been condemned as an arbitrary process. In a study of budgetting in British Columbia, it was concluded that allocations depended on the economic circumstances of the province, the requirements and character of particular hospitals, as well as the (political) relationship of the hospital with the funding agency. Attempts to inject more objective criteria of need have concentrated on 'the efficiency with which institutions are operated and changes in volume of services'. (Lewin and Associates 1976 pp. 3-24) For example, British Columbia applies normative staffing patterns; Quebec and Ontario concentrate on institutional costs. Those hospitals which deviate significantly from the expected or group norm are liable to be

investigated. Yet in practice, across-the-board
action has been found more palatable. Where changes
in service provision are requested these are usually
inspected on an itemised basis. A different
approach was adopted in Saskatchewan were 'patient
day projections' were calculated on the basis of the
population to be served. The formula included:
population served (hospital patients in individual
hospitals compared with all hospital patients
discharged from local hospitals); age-sex adjustment
(weighted for age and sex based on province wide
utilisation patterns); average days of stay
adjustment (to control for patient mix); and
adjustments for greater needs of Indians (allowance
given if the hospital serves an Indian population).
(Lewin and Associates 1976, pp. 3-28)
    The traditional method of budgetary analysis
had entailed consideration of each item separately –
'line-by-line'. In the 1970s there was a shift to
'global' budgetting in several provinces.
(Soderstrom 1978 p. 31) The argument was made that
itemised budgetting reduced the scope for local
priority setting and efficiency in accounting
procedures. The global budget provides a total
figure based on previous allocations and predicted
inflation, with additional monies for special
projects, and leaves the hospital with much more
scope to allocate these resources as it thinks best.
It does not mean that detailed budgetary submissions
are not called for prior to setting the global
amount, nor does it free the hospital from regular
reporting to ensure that it is keeping to its limit.
Again there is much inter-provincial variation.
    It is not the case that budgets fixed at the
beginning of the financial year are strictly
enforced. They are often the result of protracted
and disputed negotiation. Hence, the provincial
monitoring of hospital expenditure levels through
the year and the final adjustment are integral
elements in the budgetting system. Lewin and
Associates' Report (1976) provides an illustration
of how this process worked in British Columbia.
Initially, a 15% increase in 1974 was approved, but
this was raised to 20% during the year. This left
as many as one third of hospitals still in deficit,
but as the amounts were not deemed significant these
were met out of discretionary revenue. The province
saw this as 'deficit budgetting' in which a
deliberately tight budgetary allocation encouraged
hospital administrators to economise.
    In practice, provincial authorities have been

very loath to penalise overspending hospitals. Studies of Ontario, British Columbia and Quebec in the 1970s report on the political problems of 'bankrupting' a hospital. Provinces have therefore resorted increasingly to a carrot-and-stick approach. In both Ontario and Quebec incentive schemes have been introduced to enable hospitals to retain a specified amount of any savings, although the impact has not been significant. After ending one scheme, Ontario set out in 1982 on another attempted restructuring of hospital funding. The level of financial self-discipline was still thought unacceptable. One hundred and ten million dollars (out of a total 3.3 billion budget) was earmarked for hospitals with funding difficulties, to put them on a sound footing. After that, the government insisted that the hospitals were on their own, and had to make do with their allocation or find money from elsewhere. (Ontario 1983)

In Ontario, hospital management was provided with new opportunities under the Business Oriented New Development (BOND) programme. Introduced in 1982, it created incentives for hospital economy drives, since the hospital was allowed to retain any savings. A hospital was further encouraged to earn income additional to that provided in the provincial allocation. The encouragement of a new style of financial management in the health sector has been a developing phenomenon. Even so, few provinces have yet matched Ontario's support for private sector involvement. One sign of future developments may lie in the contract signed between an American-based hospital management corporation and an acute care hospital board in Ontario. The deal guarantees funds for a new hospital. The company will oversee the management of the hospital in order to develop budgetary savings or surpluses, whether achieved by operating efficiencies, or new revenue raising measures. The spur for the company is that, in addition to its management fee, it will take a half share of any savings. (Korcok 1983) According to press reports, the company places great emphasis on its management information programmes. These cover areas such as the discharge and transfer of patients, patient communication, doctors' orders and results, materials management and financial cost reporting. (p. 704) The anticipation is that its impact on hospital management will convince the public health sector that private business management systems and practices are able to deal with the low efficiency (and underfunding) of health services.

In Quebec, the control of acute care hospitals has been a prime target throughout the period since 1970. The means adopted include the introduction of global budgets, but it soon became apparent that deficits would be covered, and hospital costs continued to rise. So in 1974, a top-down system was introduced. Most noticeable, the government became involved in negotiating wage levels and working conditions for health workers. Hospitals in deficit were subjected to more stringent investigation, while those in surplus were offered certain incentives. Still dissatisfied, in 1976 budget increases in acute care hospitals were restricted to 2.5% (a cut in real terms), while the larger hospitals were instructed to convert at least 10% of their beds to chronic care. The planners seemed to have given up on trying to distinguish which hospitals were efficient and which were not. (Rodwin 1984 pp. 113-34) Not to be denied, health planners in the province produced the 'budgetary base review' system. This grouped hospitals 'on the basis of their diagnostic case mix and comparing their relative costs'. (p. 134) Evaluation of such attempted promotion of efficiency in terms of the effect on service provision remains uncertain. Although the measurement of programme performance, or the evaluation of the effectiveness of particular clinical practices, has not made much headway in the Canadian system, there are signs that a re-think is underway. For example, Ontario has introduced an evaluation protocol for proposed new services, such as geriatric day hospitals (Ontario 1984a). The emphasis is placed on process and outcome criteria in the fashion suggested by Donabedian (1980) although it bears close resemblance to a 'management by results and objectives' system. This heightened attention to review and evaluation mechanisms is complemented by a continuing concern with cost-efficiency. - defined in terms of 'providing the best possible care at a cost which is acceptable to individual communities and to the province as a whole'. (Ontario 1984a)

In comprison with the USA, two aspects of the budgetary process stand out: 'separation of capital and operting funds and the predominantly global nature'. (Evans 1982b p. 184) At least in their ability to control costs, Canadian hospitals have outperformed their southern neighbours. Unlike American hospitals which tend to act as independent business units, Canadian hospitals are restricted in

their operating budgets by the provincial authority,
and have less scope for independent action to
acquire expensive medical technology, or to
undertake capital projects. In further contrast,
Canadian hospital management also seems less
pressured by providers and consumers alike for the
maximum delivery of services, and thus enjoys a
'hidden saving' which is not of its making. (Aaron
and Schwartz 1984) Expenditure control and
management for the main health care providers who
are remunerated on a fee-for-service basis -
physicians and dentists - varies noticeably. The
proportion of health expenditure directed to
physicians' and dentists' services has remained
fairly steady over the years 1960-82, although the
dental expenditures per capita have been rising
faster than all other health cost categories in the
period since 1970. (Canada: Health and Welfare
1983b) The movement towards greater 'denticare'
within provincial plans has been very uneven, and in
general dental care costs have not been subject to
the same managerial scrutiny as have physicians'
services.

Fee-for-service payment, with the regular
negotiation of fee schedules provides a distinctive
context within which fiscal influences may be
employed to control both physicians' earnings and
to guide their clinical behaviour. Average net
income figures for 1971-80 indicate that physicians
have remained at the top of the professionals'
table, although the gap has narrowed. The impact of
more stringent provincial bargaining over fee-
schedules seems evident. Nevertheless, the
provincial medical associations won Medicare benefit
increases of at least 10% in every year 1980-82,
although in 1983 the increases fell to an average of
approximately 5%. This reduction reflected the
federal decision to limit public service wage
increases to 6% in 1983 and 5% in 1984, and its
exhortation to provincial governments to follow suit
in order to drastically cut inflation. Physicians
were in some cases protected from some of the
harsher measures taken against other health service
employees; in 1983, the Quebec government
legislated an 18% cut in all public service wage
rates. The controls on physicians' earnings, while
relatively effective, have not been as swingeing as
those felt in other sections of the health services,
but the containment has been sufficient to encourage
the practice of extra-billing.

Potentially, budgetary management of fee-

schedules enables the provincial authority to
stimulate more efficient and effective practices. A
weighting of fee increases or structure towards
general practitioners rather than specialists has
been a ploy used in Quebec. (Champagne et al 1983)
Equally, there is scope to influence clinical
practice. This might be an especially potent tactic
in delaying the introduction or spread of new
technologies, such as CAT scanners. The marked
increase in sclerosing injections by GPs in Quebec,
was both halted by a reduction in the fee, and re-
directed to specialists; and the growth of smear
tests was similarly controlled by including them as
part of a general consultation rather than as a
separate item. (Evans 1982b) Yet for the most part,
provinces do not seem to have involved themselves
closely with the 'internal dynamics' of the fee-
schedule, as opposed to the overall increase in fee
levels. The potential for further financial
management action remains, but for the most part, it
appears not to have seriously challenged the
entrenched occupational control enjoyed by
physicians. Not that there are obvious signs that
physicians have free rein to adapt the fee schedule
to their own financial profit. Canadians often
compare favourably their experience with that of the
United States. One possible strategy noted there
has been so-called 'fee-schedule creep' whereby a
physician can upgrade a procedure into a higher
paying category in order to improve earnings.
Quebec's experience with three types of patient
examination on the fee-schedule was that the
proportion of 'major' examinations rose
significantly, and the number of examination
categories was reduced with evident cost savings.
(Evans 1982a p. 383) Furthermore, physicians are
only paid for the services they conduct themselves.
This militates against the use of assistants to
multiply earnings. (Slayton and Trebilock 1978)
Evans (1982a) points out that in the. Canadian
system, the ability of individual physicians to set
up private laboratories to conduct diagnostic tests
is severely curtailed by the centralisation of such
services in hospitals, and in a few approved
laboratories. The potential for further managerial
action remains, but for the most part, it appears
not to have seriously challenged the occupational
control and clinical autonomy of the medical
profession. As with hospital expenditure, broad
global control strategies have been preferred, and
in the process, physicians earnings while continuing

to increase, have not mushroomed to the same extent
as in the USA. But nor has there been a determined
attempt within Canada to move physicians into more
effective clinical practices - whether validated as
such by medically defined, or other criteria. Acute
care hospitals have been told by the Canadian
Council on Hospital Accreditation to have quality
assurance programmes in operation by 1986, and it is
expected that this requirement will be extended to
other long stay institutions. (Jarvis et al 1984)
Peer review schemes which have found some favour in
the United States as yet play little part in
Canadian medical life.

MANPOWER PLANNING

The general impression left by comparative studies
of health planning is that Canadian health
authorities have not embraced planning models for
resource allocation with the speed or enthusiasm of
their counterparts in either Britain or the USA.
(Rodwin 1984) For the most part, policy making has
been reactive rather than proactive, and indicative
of a fragmented and incremental, rather than a
systematised approach. The experience of manpower
planning illustrates this conclusion very clearly.
    In its Report (1964-5), the Royal Commission on
the Health Services argued that the population to
physician ratio that then existed in Canada of 1 :
857 ought to be improved, especially as Medicare was
expected to increase demand or serve unmet needs.
It was also persuaded that physician immigration
would decrease while emigration would accelerate as
Canadian doctors sought to escape 'socialised
medicine'. In addition, population projections
suggested continued growth at existing rates. The
recommended response to these trends was for the
open. door policy for physician immigration to
continue, while four new medical schools (of the
seven proposed) were built with federal help, and
the output from existing schools was to be
increased. (Canada 1964) In a replication of
experience in Britain, the expansion of medical
school graduates was quickly implemented, but most
of the planning assumptions proved woefully wrong.
Immigration of doctors to Canada increased, and
emigration did not; the consumption of medical
services did not significantly increase as had been
forecast; and population growth eased. The outcome
was a much more substantial fall in the population

of physician ratio to 1 : 559 in 1978. At the same
time, the uneven distribution of physicians between
and within provinces still left much room for
improvement. Whereas in British Columbia the ratio
in 1978 was 1 : 528, in New Brunswick it was 1 :
890, and in the Northwest Territories (under the
control of the federal government) 1 : 1051. (p. 37
Table 11; Roos et al 1976; Beck 1973)
   This expansion in physician supply seems to run
directly counter to the professed desire to control
health costs, and governments' own analysis which
claimed that the number of physicians was the key
factor in service expansion. More medical students
and more in hospital training positions added to the
budget, but even more central was the calculation
that each new physician generated further costs
because increased medical manpower simply led to
increased consumer utilisation. (Vayda 1983; Evans
1982a, 1983)
   The response of governments has been variable.
In general, efforts have concentrated on reducing
medical school intake, as well as the number of
residency posts. Yet in British Columbia, at the
top of the physician ratio, medical student numbers
have been increased on the pretext that British
Columbia still relies too heavily on migration from
other provinces. One positive outcome of the
increase in physician supply might have been for a
more dramatic equalisation of access within
provinces as well as between them. In Newfoundland,
to illustrate the effect on the hitherto under-
doctored Atlantic provinces, ratios improved by
around 25% in the first three years of Medicare. In
other richer provinces, such as Ontario and British
Columbia, a saturation point has seemingly been
reached in the large urban areas. For example, the
latest figures for British Columbia indicate an
overall provincial ratio of 1 : 467, but in
Vancouver the figure is as low as 1 : 339, and in
Greater Victoria 1 : 360. (Canada: House of Commons
1984 no. 14; UBC 1982) The response from the health
authorities has been to tighten various rules of
practice. In many large cities, family physicians
can experience difficulties in obtaining
accreditation rights (that is, admittance for their
patients) in some hospitals. British Columbia has
introduced a scheme to refuse an insurance billing
number to physicians wishing to enter over-doctored
areas. In Quebec, recently qualified physicins are
not reimbursed to the full level of the fee-schedule
unless they set up practice in the more remote

regions of the province. Such inducements to leave the urban areas are typical of several provinces. Ontario provides incentives with grants, loans, and other perks, to encourage physicians to set up practice in remote areas. (Ontario 1983)

Medical manpower planning bears few of the hallmarks of being seriously integrated into a wider health planning process. To a large extent, the medical profession has successfully used manpower planning exercises to increase physicians numbers, and ensure that reforms strike at the 'soft targets' - immigrant doctors - and concentrate on incentives rather than sanctions. It is difficult to detect any serious movement towards re-assessment of health care roles. The experience of nurse practitioners is revealing. North of 60 degrees latitude, nurse practitioners provide a range of services which are monopolised by physicians in the rest of Canada. Substitution of nurses for physicians has been advanced as a cost-effective measure for many procedures. (Sox 1979) But in Canada nurse practitioners are still largely confined to the sub-arctic wastelands that inhibit medical representation. A second area where primary care services might effectively be taken on by non-medical personnel is suggested by experience of dental nurses in the school-based Saskatchewan Dental Plan. (Horne 1980 pp. 211-12) An evaluation of the quality of fillings and steel crowns fitted by dentists and dental nurses suggested that work completed by the latter was considered (by dental specialists from outside Saskatchewan) at least of the same standard, and generally slightly superior. The case for much greater adoption of low-cost alternatives throughut the health sector is increasingly well documented - not least in the hospital sector where health economists have argued strongly for the benefits in efficiency terms of day surgery and home care. (Horne 1980; Evans 1982b) Further claims are made about the level of 'unnecessary services', ranging from diagnostic tests to surgery. And yet the promise that 'unambiguous improvement' lies at the end of this journey has still not attracted many travellers. (Horne 1980 pp. 212-14) The explanation that many have given lies in the fee-for service system of physician remuneration, and its concentration on medical services. The process of instilling greater efficiency into the health services returns again to professional organisation and dominance.

The verdict on recent policy initiatives

designed to provide a more rational planning of
services and personnel, as well as to improve the
processes of financial management and control,
cannot be very positive. Highly complex, and
sophisticated planning strategies have not been
attractive alternatives across the ten Canadian
provinces. While experience varies in the extent of
their implementation, and in timing, the
expectations of improved efficiency and
effectiveness have been fulfilled only partially.
Unlike efficiency, effectiveness has rarely been at
centre stage in health policy making.
Nevertheless, the general pressure to increase
managerial efficiency has made in impact in holding
down the growth in health expenditure. And so far
this has been achieved without wholly alienating
consumers and health care providers.

REVIEW

Assessment of the performance of the health services
is not a recent invention, although the rapid growth
of academic studies in programme evaluation
sometimes gives that impression. Charges of
inefficiency, and poor quality pervade the history
of health care. However, with the transformation in
the organisation and funding of the health services
in Canada, evaluation has become a more pressing
issue. A central reason for this is that the health
care industry has become 'big business' - not just
economically, but in political terms as well. With
medical dominance a well-established feature,
performance evaluation of the health services brings
public interest and accountability face-to-face with
professional autonomy. As Klein (1982) further
points out significant government intervention in
the health services sows the seeds for additional
conflict between central and local obligations. In
the Canadian case, the division of responsibilities
between the federal and provincial governments has
provided ample opportunities for power struggles
over their respective evaluations of health service
performance. As a consequence, fundamental
disagreements have arisen over the objectives of the
health services (except at the most general level),
as well as in the proper criteria for measuring the
extent to which these objectives have been
achieved.
        In the immediate post-war period, the
evaluation of health services seemed less of a

dilemma. There was considerable common ground between the main 'health care players' that there should be an expansion in services. The delivery of these services was left to the professional judgement of the medical profession. The public, and political gains, lay in the much increased access to health services, and in their more equitable provision, both among social groups and between provinces.

When the expansionary phase began to wane in the late 1960s, the underlying tensions and contradictory interests surfaced. Complaints about excessive costs, inefficiency and misallocation of resources, and general mismanagement became commonplace. Governments and health service bureaucracies promoted the need for more effective planning. Performance evaluation was an adjunct to cost containment, however much it might be packaged in more rational terms. It was an attempt to impose greater external control on the main health care providers. In so doing, it largely changed the rules of the game. Until then, improvements in health status had been associated with the expansion of the health services. By the time the Lalonde Report was published in 1974, government thinking was that Canadians enjoyed a superior health care system and health status, and that the primary objective was to hold those benefits while making more efficient use of the existing level of resources. Evaluation of the health services was measured in terms of its ability to contain expenditure. But what was the guarantee that the control of health costs was not achieved at the cost of declining services? Here lay the pressure to persuade the public that the effectiveness of health services had become a primary concern. The symbolic value of such developments is clear. What is far less certain is that programme evaluation has had a noteworthy impact on health policy making.

Indeed, Canadians like to point to the popular acceptance of Medicare which, has demonstrated 'great sucess, relative to other national systems, in resource management and cost containment'. (Evans 1982b p. 190) This has been accomplished moreover, by a top down management technique which emphasises 'global limitation in the form of restraints on institutional operating budgets or new capital acquisitions, attempts to reduce numbers of health manpower, and tight negotiation of fee schedules'. (p. 190) Conversely, what the Canadian practice eschews is rigorous evaluation of the effectiveness of the health care system. While putting limits on funding, professional autonomy is allowed full play within that amount.

With rather perverse pleasure comparisons are then drawn between the Canadian success in controlling health costs and their continuing rise in the United States. While the latter country has developed a highly sophisticated set of principles for programme evaluation, Canada has talked about it, but done very little, and not seemed to suffer for all that. Nor is this to condemn the Canadian approach as 'irrational'. For so much in the health policy making process is necessarily imprecise in its objectives. Long term planning is not always the realistic option. Evaluation is set firmly in a political battle for control of the organisation and direction of the health services. The problems inherent in performance evaluation stem from the specific place and character of health services in Canadian society. This suggests the need to reassess the notion of health service performance, and to consider efficiency and effectiveness in wider social, rather than narrow organisational terms.

NOTE

1. Considerable assistance was provided to the author by many individual Canadians as well as government departments and institutions rather too numerous to mention. Special thanks must however go to Raymond Currie for making possible a visit to the University of Manitoba, to Joe Kauvert; and to the library staff at Canada House, London.

Chapter 8

THE USA: TRANSITIONS IN HEALTH SERVICES PERFORMANCE

Rockwell Schulz

The United States, with a large heterogeneous
population, has diverse and changing health services
needs and expectations. Health systems to serve
these differing needs and expectations are equally
diverse. Indeed, it is frequently stated that
United States health services are a non-system.
Certainly they are pluralistic and most certainly
they have been changing. It is important therefore
that performance be considered in the context of
those changing needs and expectations. This Chapter
will begin by briefly describing the organisation
and financing of health services in the United
States. It will then follow the sequence of
Chapters 2 to 5 by considering the concepts of
effectiveness, efficiency, acceptability and
implementation in relation to health services in the
United States. The theme for this Chapter is that
performance definitions have been changing. Until
the 1980s the emphasis has been upon effectiveness;
it is now on efficiency resulting in dramatic
changes in reimbursement incentives, organisation,
management and delivery of health services.

ORGANISATION AND FINANCE OF HEALTH SERVICES IN THE
UNITED STATES

Health services in the United States are somewhat
similar in organisation to the system prevailing in
Great Britain prior to the National Health Service.
The United States is one of the few remaining
examples in the developed world with a so called
free enterprise health system. (Roemer 1976) On the
other hand, whilst most doctors in the United States
are not on salary and have not been captive to a
universal national health insurance system, in many

respects they have less clinical autonomy than
doctors in nationalised systems such as Great
Britain. This anomaly is discussed in a later
section.

Medical care has been, and in many respects
still is, predominately a cottage industry in the
United States. The vast majority of general
practitioners, other family doctors, and specialists
(consultants), either practice alone or in single
specialty groups. About three quarters of short
term general hospitals in the United States are
private with (in 1982) 89% of private beds
controlled by not-for-profit church or other
community groups. For-profit invester owned
hospitals are a growing but still relatively small
phenomenon representing the other 11% of private
hospital beds. Almost all doctors, including
general practitioners, have privileges to admit and
treat patients in hospitals; very few are salaried
by hospitals.

Private hospitals are controlled by a governing
board consisting of church and/or community
leadership. The hospital administrator, now usually
titled 'president', is responsible to the board for
all hospital personnel including nurses, physical
facilities and finances. Doctors on the other hand
are independent and essentially clients of the
hospital, but subject to bylaws, rules and
regulations of their own medical staff organisation.
The hospital organisation has been referred to as a
duopoly with separate hospital and medical staff
organisations which relate to each other either
through a joint conference committee or, increasingly, through a medical director. (Schulz and
Johnson 1983) Although the medical staff is
organisationally separate, the hospital governing
board has power of granting admission privileges to
medical staff members based on the recommendations
of the medical staff credentials committee. Moreover, the board is legally responsible for quality
of care within the hospital, and to be accredited
(see below) must ensure that there is an effective
quality assurance program. In essence therefore,
individual doctors in the United States have more
clinical accountability to the medical staff
organisation, administrator and governing board than
consultants in Britain have to their peers, District
authorities or managers. (Schulz and Harrison 1983)

Most health services are organised privately in
the United States; nevertheless, financing of health
services is collectivised through government or

private programmes. For example, 42% of health care costs are financed by government sources mainly through Medicare (a federal universal social security health insurance mainly for persons over 65 years of age), Medicaid (a state and federally funded programme for indigent persons), and to some extent by other state and local government sources. Private funding too is collectised, primarily through employer health insurance plans, such as the not-for-profit Blue Cross for hospital care and Blue Shield for doctor services, or the for-profit commercial carriers. Nearly 92% of the population has some medical coverage through third party payments such as the above. However, only 70% of costs are paid by third party payers, the balance being direct payment by patients. For the most part, at least up to the mid-1980s, doctors and hospitals are reimbursed on a retrospective fee-for-service basis. That is, they bill the patient or third party for whatever services were rendered to the patient, based primarily on costs for hospital services, and reasonable and customary physician charges for that area. In 1984, however, the Federal Medicare and Medicaid programmes implemented a prospective payment system (PPS) based on diagnosis related groupings (DRGs) for hospital reimbursement, and a number of states were moving in the same direction for all hospital payers. Many expect that doctors too will eventually be reimbursed prospectively for Medicare and Medicaid services or on a capitation basis through Health Maintenance Organisations (HMOs).

Although most medical services are private, there are a number of national health service systems operating. The first was organised in the 18th century for American seamen and was the forerunner of the United States Public Health Service. The Veterans Administration operates a large national health service for armed forces veterans, which represents nearly 2% of all hospital beds in the United States. A small but unique model for delivering comprehensive health promotion as well as medical services to help meet the broad health needs of the urban and rural poor is the Community Health Centre programme of which there were 112 such centres in the United States in 1978. There is another example of a nationally funded system, which provides comprehensive mental health services. Finally, over 20% of short term general and other special hospital beds are owned by state and local governments. Among these are the large

local government funded public charity type
hospitals in many of the largest urban centres. The
Medicaid programme for the poor was expected to make
such hospitals obsolete by providing indigents with
a means for paying for care in private hospitals.
However, with current reductions in federal
programmes for indigents, patient loads at the large
charity public hospitals are again increasing.
Interestingly, many of the local government public
hospitals are contracting with private management
firms to operate those hospitals on their behalf.

Over the years there has been agitation for
universal national health insurance and even a
national health service in United States. In 1917
the American Medical Association argued for a
national health insurance, but in 1922 rescinded
this position and since then has strongly and
effectively lobbied against such proposals. With
the recent rising costs of medical care, increasing
federal deficits and the current conservative
government, little is heard about nationalising
health services or their financing. In summary, the
United States health system is diverse; a general
review of its performance is therefore difficult.
In evaluating its performance this Chapter focuses
mainly on the largest sector, the non-governmental
health service systems, except where otherwise
noted.

EFFECTIVENESS OF HEALTH SERVICES IN THE UNITED
STATES

While the desired effect of health services, that
is, to improve health, has not changed, expectations
for achieving that goal have changed considerably.
Insofar as mortality can be taken as a proxy for
morbidity, health status in the United States has
improved as it has worldwide as evidenced by
declining death rates and increasing longevity.
McDermott (1969) suggested there were four stages of
medicine:

> Stage 1: Impersonal measures that result in
> better health such as eating from a
> table instead of a dirty floor,
> improvements in roads and other means
> of transportation and communication,
> etc.

Stage 2: Environmental health measures such as safe water supply, use of insecticides to control malaria, etc.

Stage 3: Public health measures such as immunisation programmes.

Stage 4: Personal health measures, especially physician intervention.

Each of these stages has been grafted onto the next. Stages 1, 2, and 3 are still important today since the influence of transportation, pollution, vaccinations for measles and polio etc. on health is recognised. Stage 4 measures really become effective in the mid-1920s and 1930s; it is the stage when modern medical technology became decisive and more effective. Prior to Stage 4, according to McDermott, physicians provided only human comfort. He suggests that Stage 4 coincides with the introduction of antimicrobial drugs. Continuing progress, such as substantial improvements in treatment of cancer, is evident as Stage 4 continues along with the other stages.

A Stage 5, beginning in the 1980s might be added to McDermott's four stages and be labelled:

Stage 5: Self-care such as exercise, diet, risk reductions, self-help groups and potentially computer assisted self-diagnosis and primary treatment services.

Before describing Stage 5 it is necessary to examine intervening years from the 1960s to the 1980s. In the 1960s, the performance of health services in the United States was defined in structural and process terms. (Donabedian 1980) The objective of the health system during Stage 4 was the advancement and especially the application of medical knowledge. National policy for achieving this objective was to expand the structure and provide resources for advances and to establish processes to ensure that the advanced knowledge was applied. With an expanding economy the federal government injected billions of dollars into medical research. The delivery structure also expanded with the introduction of federal funds to increase the number and size of hospitals (the Hill-Burton programme which begin in 1946) and massive support for the education of physicians and of other health professions in order to increase the health manpower pool. Access to an enlarged medical care structure also increased through the implementation in 1966 of a national health insurance system for the elderly (Medicare) and a state and national shared programme to enable indigents to obtain private medical services (Medicaid). Also during the Kennedy and Johnson presidential eras, the federal Community Mental Health Centre and Neighborhood (Community) Health Centre Programmes were planned and implemented. Consistent with the health services objectives defined above, the Regional Medical programme was also established in 1965 (but phased out in the 1970s) to conquer heart, stroke and and cancer by spreading advanced medical technologies from university medical centres through regional systems.

Process as well as structural measures were taken to improve the effectiveness of health services in the United States. Historically, general practitioners as well as specialists have had hospital admitting privileges. To ensure quality of care, a voluntary non-governmental accreditation system the Joint Commission of Accreditation of Hospitals (JCAH) began in the 1950s as an outgrowth of a predecessor organisation started by the American College of Surgeons before 1920. To become accredited the JCAH requires hospitals to evaluate the quality of care and define physician privileges. JCAH has considerable influence in that accredited hospitals with utilisation review programmes are automatically certified for reimbursement under Medicare. In 1973 the physician evaluation (peer review) system was expanded with the implementation of 'Professional Standards Review Organisations' (PSROs now called Professional Review Organisations [PRO]), to ensure the quality of care and appropriate use of services for Medicare and Medicaid patients. The JCAH and PRO mandated quality review systems require an audit review of inpatient medical records to ensure that processes of care are of high quality and really necessary.

However, beginning in the 1970s the focus has been on outcomes as well as processes. Authors such as Illich (1975), McKeown (1976) and Carlson (1975) raised questions about the effectiveness of medical care services in improving health of populations and persons. McKeown suggests that past improvements in health services must be attributed largely to public health and environmental influences, whilst Illich

and survival rates there is considerable evidence of
continuing improvements. The age-adjusted death
rate in the United States has dropped from nearly 13
deaths per thousand population in 1930 to less than
6 in 1980. Since 1968 there has been a drop in death
rates for 12 of the 15 major killers. The death
rate for heart disease decreased 25% between 1970
and 1982, and 40% for strokes during the same
period. Infant mortality has shown a steady decline
while at the other end of the age spectrum age
adjusted death rates for the elderly declined 27%
between 1950 and 1979. Life expectancy rose to a
new high in 1982 at 74.5 years, but life expenctancy
for women was over 7 years beyond men, and for
whites, 6 years beyond blacks. However, the gap is
narrowing as life expectancy for black Americans
increased 5.2 years from 1970 to 1982 compared with
3.4 years for whites. Nevertheless health status
disparities remain between education, income and
ethnic groups as they do in Britain, and of course
it is far from clear that the improvements described
above can be attributed to changes in health
services.

EFFICIENCY OF HEALTH SERVICES IN THE UNITED STATES

Discussion of health services effficency in the
United States has not always been conducted in
consistent language. For example, the term
'efficiency' has been used in a way different from
any of those described in Chapter 3 above; Pauly
(1972 pp. 3-4) defines technical efficiency as
follows:

> Standards of 'high quality' or 'good' medical
> care are set in the light of current medical
> practice and inefficiency exists when care in
> excess of or in any way differing from these
> standards is provided ... waste therefore
> occur(s) when current methods are not used.
> Little reference is made to individual demands
> or tastes for various types of care, and there
> is no attempt to compare costs of such care
> with the evaluations its recipients make of
> it.

On such a definition, health services in the USA
must be considered to have become increasingly
technically efficient.
Moving to other concepts of efficiency, in

The United States of America

terms of distributive efficiency considerable
progress has been made toward equity in access.
Nearly 92% have health insurance and the utilisation
of services among the poor and blacks is now greater
than among upper income and white persons. Before
the implementation of Medicare and Medicaid,
physician visits per person were substantially below
for both groups. Nevertheless, perhaps the poor
should be receiving more care, and nearly 20 million
persons in the United States in 1982 were without
insurance. There are also persons who are
underinsured and may not be receiving adequate care.
While there may still be some financial barriers to
equal access, system growth and reimbursement
incentives removed queues to service and have
removed barriers such as age to such services as
renal dialysis and hip replacements, which are
rationed or inaccessible to many elderly in Britain.
(Aaron and Schwartz 1984)

If one examines managerial efficiency (the
production process which for a given level of output
minimizes the cost of inputs to produce that
output), the United States falls far short. Macrae
(1984 p. 18) suggests that Britain and Japan in
particular exceed the United States in managerial
efficiency. Macrae argues that the 'lowest input
brings best output' though he assumes that health
expenditure and the number of doctors relate to
health status, ignoring the role of genetic
endowment, enviroment, nutrition and behaviours
which have a much greater impact on health status
indicators. (Schulz and Johnson 1983) It also
ignores the role that medicine plays in improving
the quality of life of individual. Moreover, when
one examines health status within comparable socio-
economic groups, health status indicators between
countries are more similar.

Medical expenditure in the United States
increased to over 10% of the Gross National Product
in 1982. However, until the 1980s the rapid rise
in health care costs in the United States was felt
seriously only by federal and state governments,
which rely on taxation to support health services.
In the past, employers could easily pass on
increased costs in the price of goods sold. Fee-
for-service, cost based reimbursement has been
regarded as a sacred tradition in American medicine.
The American Medical Association and its doctor
constituents have long held that effective doctor-
patient relationships are best obtained, (along with
doctor earnings) when the patient can select

whichever doctor he or she prefers, and pays the
doctor directly (or through an insurance policy); in
these circumstances, it is considered that doctor
responsiveness to patient demands and needs is
enhanced. This position is not inconsistent with
American 'free enterprise' traditions.

While there may be some merit to this, as noted
in Chapter 3, medical care is however, a classic
example of market failure. Until 1984 even federal
programmes of Medicare and Medicaid were based on
this freedom of choice, fee-for-service principle.
Through Medicare, Medicaid or other health insurance
the doctor could be assured of reimbursement for
whatever 'reasonable and customary charges' were
incurred to treat a patient, and hospitals
reimbursed at their costs. This cost based
reimbursement provided incentives to apply latest
knowledge and technology, that is, the highest
quality of care. Full cost reimbursement for most
patients at the same time provided incentives for
patients to demand maximum service. Cost based
reimbursement was also an incentive to doctors and
hospitals to increase the use and cost of services,
because increased costs increased income. Only the
government had problems passing such costs on to
others. In other words, there were really no
incentives for efficiency in the United States
health services.

Relying on their regulatory powers, federal and
state governments enacted a number of laws in
attempts to ensure efficiency. In 1946 with the
enactment of the Hill-Burton hospital construction
programme, the federal government initiated its
involvement in the health system in a major way when
it required a state survey of a need for health
facilities and a plan for meeting those needs. In
1966 with the beginning of Medicare and Medicaid
Public Law (P L) 89-749, Comprehensive Health
Planning (CHP) extended health facilities planning
and co-ordination, but still on a voluntary basis.
In the mid-1970s there were a number of legislative
actions that attempted to rationalise the system and
to control costs. In 1973 P L 92-603 established
PSROs and Section 1122 further strengthened planning
when it required hospitals to obtain a 'Certificate
of Need' (CON) from local and state planning
agencies for any major facility expansion or
replacement. The 1974 National Health Planning and
Resource Development Act (P L 93-641) consolidated
and attempted to strengthen federal programmes by
replacing planning with regulation.

The United States of America

Rapidly rising costs of the Medicaid programme, for which the states are required to share costs, prompted a number of states to implement prospective rate review programmes. Except in a handful of states which had more Draconian rate review regulations, neither state nor federal regulatory efforts have ameliorated rising costs in the United States.

Continuing increases in health care costs at more than double the inflation rate of the rest of the economy, projected bankruptcy of Medicare, high federal budget deficits and a major recession called for new health care priorities and measures in the mid-1980s. Efficiency took precedence over effectiveness especially when there was increasing concern regarding the benefits of some new health care technologies. In 1980 with the inauguration of Ronald Reagan as President there was a rebirth of free enterprise conservatism in the United States. Furthermore, based on prior experience there was evidence that regulation merely protected the interests of those whom the system was designed to regulate in that it protected hospital markets and prevented hospital failures and closures. (Colby and Begley 1983) Economists such as Enthoven in the late 1970s and early 1980s articulated competition as a way to control medical costs. (Enthoven 1978) About that time a group of health services researchers at Yale University developed a method of classifying patients by diagnosis. Though originally unintended by the researchers, DRGs provided a way to characterise different case mixes to reimburse hospitals prospectively by paying a set rate for a specific diagnosis. Prospective Payment System (PPS) for Medicare and Medicaid patients provided incentives to contain costs in order to increase income rather than increase costs as had been the case under a cost reimbursement system. In other words, by paying a specific rate for a patient in a specific DRG the hospital could earn a profit on that patient if it cost less to treat the patient, or lose if it cost more. Although there is less than one year's experience with PPS, it is already evident that lengths of stay have fallen substantially and that hospitals are containing costs by increasing productivity resulting in increasing numbers of nurses and other employees becoming redundant.

Further pressure on costs came from the fact that in the 1980s American industry discovered that it was substantially less competitive in world

markets and it could no longer pass on increasing
health benefit costs to consumers. The Chrysler
Corporation, for example, which survived bankruptcy
by a federal government bail-out, found that health
care benefits for current and retired employees
added $600 to the price of its automobiles in 1983.
Many businesses therefore required employees to pay
a part of their medical service charges thereby
placing incentives on them not to use such services.
Part of the decline in hospital use can be
attributed to cost sharing and patient incentives
for less utilisation. A major RAND corporation
study found that cost sharing by patients reduces
utilisation without adverse effects on health
status. (Newhouse et al 1982)

Health Maitenance Organisations (HMOs) and
Preferred Provider Organisations (PPOs) are other
mechanisms used by employers to provide
reimbursement incentives on doctors to contain
costs. The Kaiser-Permanente health system based in
California provided the model for HMO organisations
many years ago, while Paul Elwood of Minnesota
coined the phrase and was instrumental in promoting
HMOs. There are three categories of HMOs: firstly,
the 'staff model' where a consumer governing board
employs doctors on a salary arrangement as in the
successful Group Health Plans in a number of cities.
Secondly there is the 'group model' where doctors
own the group and contract with the HMO plan to
provide medical services as in the Kaiser Health
Plan. Thirdly the 'Independent Practice Plan (IPA)
model' is where doctors are independent in solo or
small group practice and do not pool expenses as in
the group model. Many county medical societies
sponsor IPAs, usually on an open panel plan basis
where any doctor can join, though in some cases a
closed panel plan where doctors are selected to
join. HMOs are prepaid health plans; in other
words, doctors are paid an annual fee on a
capitation basis to provide health services for a
defined population. Financial incentives to HMO
doctors are to maintain a person's health so he or
she will not require costly medical care services,
hence the reference to 'health maintenance'. In
fee-for-service plans the more service a doctor
provides, that is, the higher the costs, the more
the doctor will earn. In HMOs the doctor receives
his fee at the beginning of the year for all
services, therefore the lower the hospital and
other costs, the more the doctor will earn.
Experience has shown that costs in group and staff

model HMOs are 10% to 40% lower than fee-for-service
plans, primarily attributable to doctors' methods of
practice which utilise less hospital inpatient
service. (Manning et al 1984) There has been no
evidence that open panel IPAs, which exercise little
control over doctors, have achieved significant
savings over fee-for-service plans.

Preferred Provider Organisations (PPOs) are
another reimbursement model aimed at promoting
competition and cost containment incentives. PPO
plans contract with doctors and hospitals for a
discount - usually around 25% - to Plan members.
PPO enrollees consequently pay nothing or little if
they use a PPO, or they pay the difference between
the discounted and full charge if they do not use
the PPO.

A growing surplus of doctors and hospital
services has encouraged HMO and PPO models.
Minneapolis/St. Paul, Minnesota and Madison,
Wisconsin have been especially active in the
adoption of HMOs with about one third of the
Minnesota cities' population enrolled in HMOs and an
even higher percentage enrolled in HMOs in Madison.
There is preliminary evidence in both these areas
that HMOs help to contain costs.

In summary, it is necessary to consider
changing approaches to efficiency. Until nearly the
1980s so-called technical efficiency was the major
standard in the United States. Objectives were to
obtain resources to meet rising demands to apply
advancing medical processes to all persons in need
of care; the system was inefficient if such
processes were not applied. From 1966 onwards, this
was combined with a concern for distributive
efficiency. Today, the standards are managerial
efficiency, that is, to produce healthy outcomes at
least cost. The federal government has provided
massive support to advance knowledge, expand the
system to apply it, and provide resources to the
elderly and needy to purchase such medical
technology, but in 1984 a near revolution has
occurred in the medical care system to shift it from
a cost based reimbursement to a prospective and
capitation system in order to meet new priorities
for managerial efficiency. Only meagre anecdotal
evidence is available at this time, but it appears
that the system is responding to those revised
objectives.

EFFECTIVENESS AND EFFICIENCY

How do effectiveness and efficiency relate to each
other? As noted in Chapter 3 above, efficiency most
appropriately utilises effectiveness in its
objective for maximisation. An important issue
therefore is whether or not higher quality care
relates to higher costs. Conventional wisdom might
suggest that it does. On the other hand, Macrae
(1984) suggests that lower costs relates to higher
quality in terms of outcomes. Although Scott et al
(1979) in an evaluation of surgical mortality rates
found higher costs per hospital day related to
survival, Shortell et al (1976) found that lower
costs per hospital stay related to higher quality in
terms of severity adjusted mortality rates among
hospitals he studied. Schulz, Greenley and Peterson
(1983) found cost and perceived quality in thirteen
acute inpatient psychiatric units were related to
goal preferences of units and management practices
employed to achieve those goals. As Figure 8.1
indicates, they found a wide range of cost per case
and indicators of quality with some units having low
costs and high quality, others low costs but low
quality, others high quality but high costs and some
both high costs and low quality. These outcomes
were not related to environment, patient,
institutional or professional practice
characteristics; their relationships to management
practices are discussed in the final section of this
Chapter.

Figure 8.1: Relationship of Cost Per Case and
Quality Among 13 Acute Inpatient Psychiatric Units

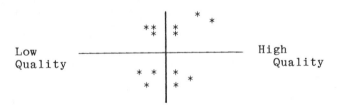

Low Cost Per Case

Low
Quality

High
Quality

High Cost Per Case

Adapted from Schulz, Greenley and Peterson (1983)
and reproduced by permission from Medical Care.

ACCEPTABILITY

Whether or not something is acceptable and how
acceptable it is will relate to expectations. If a
person expects access to medical care, it is
unacceptable not to receive it. If a person
expects that medicine can cure he is likely to
pursue a medical cure until proven wrong, or until
the patient and family are convinced all that is
medically possible has been done. As noted in
Chapter 4 acceptability ranges from tolerance to
pleasure. What is considered acceptable medical
care by the British public may be unacceptable in
the United States and vice-versa. For example, a
nine month or longer wait for a hip replacement may
be tolerably acceptable in Britain, but it would be
unacceptable in the United States. A patient aged
65 in Britain with a fatal kidney disease may accept
a doctor's statement that nothing can be done, while
in the United States renal dialysis would be
demanded. On the other hand, an individual
bedridden with pain and a high fever in Britain
would find it unacceptable for a doctor not to make
a house call, while in the United States such a
person would expect to get out of bed and arrange
some way to get to the doctor's office or hospital
if he felt medical attention was needed. The
American would be very pleased, however, if the
doctor did make a house call because he would not
have expected it. It is interesting to note that
doctors are just now beginning again to make house
calls in the United States as there is a growing
surplus of doctors and increasing competition for
patients between doctors.
The acceptability of medical care is also
transitional. Before Phase 4 (decisive medicine),
little was expected of medicine in the way of cure,
consequently home remedies, prayer, other non-
technological methods and the doctor's emotional
support were acceptable. During Phase 4, people
expected medicine to cure. As we enter Phase 5,
more people expect a selfcare-medical care
partnership approach to maximum health and illness
cure. Unacceptability therefore is the gap between
the expected and the actual. Consumers, providers
and payers have different priorities in expectations
and definitions of acceptability.
Thus consumers expect access to medical care,
that it has a reputation for high quality, that they
are treated with humaneness and that it is
affordable. Doctors on the other hand are likely

to see priorities in applying their advanced knowledge and skills with high quality services, in maintaining their autonomy to do so, and in being appropriately rewarded for their sacrifices to obtain and practice their advanced knowledge and skills. Payers, as might be expected, have priorities related to cost of care.

Consumers in the United States as in Britain appear generally pleased with their own medical care services. People in Britain will remark how difficult it must be for people to become ill in America and become bankrupt to pay for care if they can afford to seek it all, while Americans will remark how difficult it must be to need care in the 'socialised' British system with low quality service. Neither generalisation is of course accurate. In many respects with full insurance coverage and cost based reimbursement there is greater access to care in the United States, while Americans equate quality with newness of facilities even though consultants in Britain have more extensive training than many doctors in American hospitals.

Public opinion polls play a major role in the way of life in the United States from its elective government bodies to the market oriented economy. Such polls have consistently shown people to be generally very pleased with their own access, quality and cost of medical services and yet critical of the system. In a 1983 Harris Poll, only 21% expressed the belief that the United States's health care system 'works pretty well' (Iglehart 1984). Turning to the attitudes of providers, doctors in the United States have focussed on quality as a means of improving acceptability of care, that is, the application of advancing medical knowledge and skills. As noted above, quality assurance activities have centred on the process of care, with an elaborate peer review system as mandated by JCAH and PROs. While Van T'Hoff (1981) reports there is little formal peer review such as medical audits of medical and surgical services in Britain, virtually all hospitals in the United States have medical audit. Williams and Brook (1978) reported in 1978 that quality review activities and continuing medical education have resulted in expenditure of over $1 billion annually, and if vigorously pursued will consume more than two percent of the medical care dollar. In a study of five different methods of processes and outcome evaluations Brook and Appel (1973) found that

quality of care depended on the evaluation method
used. For 296 patients reviewed in a major city
hospital, from 1.4% to 63.2% of the patients were
judged to have received adequate care depending upon
the method used to evaluate quality of patient care.
Judgement of process using explicit criteria
yielded the fewest acceptable cases, while outcome
measures yielded the most. With so much effort
expended upon quality assurance, one must assume
that doctors find quality to be at least acceptable
and perhaps professionally very satisfying.
However, less than half (48%) of all doctors
according to the 1984 Harris Poll believe that the
American health care system works well and needs
only minor chages. This is more than twice the
percentage of consumers who think it works well.
There was no consensus among physicians with regard
to priorities for change. Changes related to better
access would be given top priority by 20%, 14% cited
changes related to cost containment and 14% of the
doctors would favour less government interference
and regulation.

It can be hypothesised that clinical autonomy
would be a major source of satisfaction to
physicians, although its acceptability will vary by
type and location of practice. Doctors in solo
practice and those in more isolated rural areas
prize independence and autonomy more than doctors in
group practice, where professional stimulation is
seen as more important than autonomy. A 1984
(Scheckler and Schulz forthcoming) survey of 842
doctors in Dane County, Wisconsin (population about
325,000 with a relatively high socio-economic
status) found the priorities, set out in Table 8.1.

These priorities were also analysed by primary
care, specialist and hospital based doctors, but no
significant differences were found. A survey in
England found that freedom from formal review was
considered much more important than in the USA
(Harrison, Pohlman and Mercer forthcoming).

Rewards for arduous training and the cost of
education are obviously satisfying to doctors as
evidenced by the large number of students applying
to medical schools. Typically specialists will be
about 30 years old and considerably in debt before
they obtain their own practice. However, average
income of surgical specialists in 1982 was over
$130,000. The average work week for all doctors was
52 hours in 1982, down from 60 hours in 1958.
Opinion polls also show that doctors are among the

Table 8.1: Dane County, Wisconsin Doctors' Reported Priorities for Clinical Autonomy (n = 497)

	Very Important	Important	Unimportant	Very Unimportant
1. Freedom to order whatever you believe will help the patients	65%	33%	1%	0%
2. Patient's freedom to choose a doctor	61	34	3	1
3. Freedom to decide which services nurses can and should provide to patients	27	53	14	3
4. Doctors freedom to charge whatever they believe is reasonable	15	53	22	6
5. Doctors freedom to reject patients for non clinical reasons	7	39	24	9
6. Freedom to ignore costs of care when treating patients needs	9	41	31	16
7. Freedom from peer review audit	2	7	46	42

Reproduced from Scheckler and Schulz (1984), by permission of the authors

highest esteemed of all occupations in the United
States. Hospital administrators, have also risen in
status and income as hospitals have increased in
size and complexity.

Do doctors and consumers have the same
expectations? Scheckler and Schulz (1984) obtained
responses from about 1,000 consumers who were State
of Wisconsin employees regarding which of the
factors listed in Table 8.2 were most important to
them in selecting their primary source of care.
Dane County physicians were asked how important they
thought each of those same factors were to their
patients. The Table shows that medical competence,
range of services available, convenience, cost to
patients, chance of referrals, and which hospital
the doctors use were more important to consumers
than doctors believed they were.

Finally, it should be noted that health care
costs have become unacceptable to employers as well
as governments in recent years. Formerly, employers
capitulated to union demands for comprehensive
medical care benefits. Health insurance has been a
tax free benefit to employees. In the 1980s
businesses in the United States are less able to
pass on costs in the price of goods sold, and
consequently costs and incentives are being shifted
to employees through co-payments and deductables and
to providers through competitive HMO and PPO
bidding. Regulation of health care services failed
to achieve acceptable cost levels and it remains to
be seen if PPS will achieve them or if further
actions will be necessary. At any rate dramatic
changes in the funding, organisation and delivery of
health services in the United States are resulting
from the unacceptability of rising costs of health
care services to government and employer payers.
However, as cost containment criteria begin to
dominate, it seems possible that access to care and
its quality will become less acceptable or at least
less satisfying to both consumers and providers.
Nevertheless, taking a longer range historical
view it appears that while there may currently be
dissatisfaction with the system as a whole as it is
in the process of dramatic change, health services
in the United States have been acceptable to most
individuals. Given the evidence that increasing
managerial efficiency does not necessarily result in
less effective services there is hope for some kind
of accommodation to current financial pressures. As
Aaron and Schwartz (1984 p. 133 ff) note however, it
is the continuing development of health care

Table 8.2: Importance of Various Factors to Consumers in Selecting Primary Source of Health Care Compared With Doctors Perceptions of What They Think are Patients Preferences

1) Consumers (n = 1062)
2) Doctors (n = 497)

	Very Important (1)	Important (2)	Sub Total	Unimportant (3)	Very Unimportant (4)
Availability of care when needed	1) 85% 2) 83	13% 16	98% 99	– –	0 0
Medical competence	1) 92 2) 71	7 21	99 92	– 5	– –
Treatment as a person and an individual	1) 64 2) 69	32 29	96 98	2 1	0 0
Range of services available	1) 62 2) 31	34 58	96 89	2 9	– –
Convenience of location	1) 38 2) 11	48 62	86 73	12 23	– 2
Cost to patient	1) 56 2) 32	39 61	95 93	3 5	– 0
Cost to patient's employer	1) 20 2) 20	48 41	68 61	16 23	4 13
Opportunity to see the same doctor	1) 58 2) 39	33 55	91 94	6 5	– –
Chance of referrals to other doctors	1) 61 2) 34	34 55	95 89	2 8	– –
Which hospital the doctor uses	1) 30 2) 10	41 49	71 59	23 33	2 6
Availability of evening hours	1) 13 2) 5	29 45	42 50	44 44	5 3

– = greater than 0 but less than 1%

Reproduced from Scheckler and Schulz (1984), by permission of the authors technologies which will lead to some painful rationing decisions.

IMPLEMENTATION: WHO DETERMINES PERFORMANCE AND HOW?

Health services in the United States can best be understood in terms of a combination of the external control and and pluralistic models set out in Chapter 5. The system consists of a wide range of actors whose relative influence is affected by changes over time in the environment. The Flexner Report (1910) which signalled a training response to the beginning of Phase 4 (decisive medicine) articulated a need for change in medical education and service toward scientific and university based disciplinary knowledge. Medicine became effective in intervening on the course of illness. Medical schools which Flexner patterned after the Johns Hopkins model have been a continuing influence with their control of knowledge through training and research.

Evolving change in control over financial resources has influenced or reflected implementation of health care service changes. Until about the 1920s and 1930s philanthropists who donated funds for hospitals and other health services and consequently controlled them had the dominating influence. From the 1930s into the 1960s doctors controlled not only knowledge, but financial resources through patient fee-for-service payments. In the 1960s and 1970s hospital managers increased their power when doctors became more dependent on the hospital as their workshop and hospitals bargained with third party payers for resources. In the late 1970s the corporate form of medicine burgeoned as invester owned for-profit hospitals developed and expanded rapidly, and not-for-profit hospitals formed multi-institutional arrangements and systems. In the 1980s the federal government and employers, in a crisis of rising health care costs and diminishing resources, exercised their power by changing incentives from retrospective to prospective reimbursement systems. Environmental changes are also giving consumers increasing power to implement change. With the supply of doctors and hospitals exceeding demand, both are becoming more market oriented to attract patients. Meanwhile through Preferred Provider Organisations and Health Maintenance Organisations, consumers have collective bargaining power to implement provider changes. An

example is the development of staff model HMOs
whereby consumer boards employ doctors on a salary
and bargain with competing hospitals for favourable
prices and services. Furthermore, if self care
trends continue, consumers will have more influence
over their own care as well as the system design.

Health services in the United States are
basically pluralistic and seem likely to remain so
for the forseeable future. There have been any
number of attempts to reduce this pluralism through
at least a compulsory national insurance scheme, but
with rising costs and federal budget deficits, it is
unlikely that it will be implemented unless the
fiscal crisis becomes so great that the system is
nationalised to gain control. One might debate
whether or not the system is satisficing and
reactive as suggested in bounded rational models,
but providers have historically been proactive and
payers and consumers increasingly so. Starr (1982)
suggests that the pluralistic model in the United
States has been 'elitist' with doctors dominating
through most of recent history. However, with
growing influence by payers and consumers, power
seems fairly widely disbursed today. While Starr
proposes that organised medicine in the United
States has historically managed the system to
protect medical sovereignty, it is interesting to
compare clinical autonomy of doctors in the United
States with autonomy of British clinicians. Since
the 1920s doctors in the United States have
vehemently resisted national health service or
insurance in order to protect their independence.
They have maintained ownership of their practice and
profits therefrom. However, in actual freedom to
order services they desire for their patients, they
appear to have less autonomy than their British
colleagues. In maintaining the privileges of
general practitioners to admit and treat patients in
hospitals, an elaborate peer review system has been
established which defines what a doctor can and
cannot do in a hospital. Moreover, in efforts to
contain costs there is a utilisation review system
which evaluates and controls admissions, services
ordered and length of hospital stay. These control
systems whilst no doubt improving quality and
containing costs, limit freedom of individual
doctors to treat as they may want. Their British
consultant counterparts by contrast have
relinquished ownership and income, but retained
practice freedoms in accepting the NHS. Which
system protects patient interests best or what other

The United States of America

system might do it better is debatable.

CONCLUDING OBSERVATIONS

The health service system in the United States, and
its performance, are dynamic and result from a
combination of changing forces. It has been, and
continues to be, shaped by a changing social,
technological, and economic environment in which it
functions. It is also shaped by actors in the
system including providers of care, government
policy makers and other payers, the legal system,
institutional managers, and consumers. In the final
sub-sections the influence of each of these to date
and expectations for the future are considered.

Environmental Influence
While analysts tend to focus on the actors in the
system, the environment in which the system operates
also has great influence in defining efficiency and
effectiveness and its performance in relation to
definitions. The United States is one of the
wealthiest nations in the world today and it clings
to its pioneer individualistic heritage. The health
system mirrors the nation's economic, social and
technological environment. Until the 1980s it has
been a growing industry in a growing economy
applying advancing technology similar to other high
technology industries. In the Kennedy-Johnson
social revolution of the 1960s, health services were
extended to the previously deprived. With the re-
emergence of conservatism expressed in the Reagan
administration along with a shrinking economy for
social welfare programmes, health services
competition and industrialistion arise.
    In the current fragile national and
international political, economic and social
environment, it is hard to predict the future.
However, resources available for health care are
liable to continue to shrink causing further
contraction of the system. There is little reason
to expect an abatement of technological advances,
but rising costs of technology will further strain
providers in implementing these. An ageing
population will add to needs for service, while
advancing educational levels of consumers will raise
their self care capabilities and their knowledge
about, and hence demand for, treatment. The economy
will force increased efficiency and cost

219

containment. Values are likely to continue to change as well, and one might predict a shift back towards preferences for equity (distributive efficiency) in health service consumption away from current libertarian individualism. Providers, policy makers and payers, the legal system, managers and patients will have to adapt to such continuing changes.

Provider Influence

Doctors have historically dominated health services by setting professional standards for health care. Their power to dominate stems from a variety of sources such as unquestioned expertise, patient loyalties, elitist qualifications to enter medical school, influence over hospital resources, and standard setting by professional organisations such as the American Medical Association. While doctors in the United States enjoy high status similar to their British counterparts, their favoured economic position has tarnished public sympathies for them, and no doubt contributed to a recent lessening of their influence over the definition of efficiency. The environment changes described above are likely to change definitions of efficiency, effectiveness and acceptability. They certainly will change the provider delivery system. However, in relation to today's emphasis on efficiency, continuing improvements can be expected. Medical care in the United States is likely to move from a cottage industry into a relatively few competing health care systems. Whereas a few years ago the community general hospitals in the United States were relatively autonomous units, today one third are operated by multi-hospital systems. It has been projected that as those hospitals which survive economic constraints join systems, and hospital systems themselves merge, there may be fewer than 100 systems compared with the 7,000 relatively autonomous institutions in the past. Furthermore, as doctors merge into groups to provide HMO or PPO services they may merge or more closely affiliate with hospital systems as well. Older doctors comfortable in solo or small group practices find such changes frightening, but younger doctors facing a projected physician glut will adjust. Should competitive market models not achieve currently prevailing concepts of efficiency, nationalised health services may be seen as a logical alternative for government control over costs. Thus one way or

another medical care is likely to organise into
large systems. Control is more direct over
centralised systems than cottage industries, and in
the process of control, formalised effectiveness and
efficiency standards, measures and reward systems
will develop.

Policy Maker and Payer Influence

Policy makers and payers who provide resources and
incentives to providers have had a growing influence
over health care service performance. Beginning
with licensing, then providing capital, manpower
training, funding, and more recently introducing
regulation and reimbursement incentives, government
policy makers have influenced the effectiveness,
efficiency and acceptability of health services in
the United States. However, whilst policy makers
may have properly diagnosed needs for performance
improvements in the system, implementation of
policies has lagged so far behind needs, that they
have at times been counterproductive. For example,
it was probably clear to policy makers at the end of
World War II that health manpower, especially
doctors, would be seriously short for a growing
population, yet funding to expand training was not
implemented until the 1960s. Consequently with the
long lead time to construct training facilities,
staff them and train doctors, by the time production
reached its peak in the late 1970s and early 1980s,
needs changed and priorities for cost containment
called for health system and manpower reductions.
At this time in the mid 1980s with doctors finding
practice opportunities increasingly scarce, there is
still little evidence of health manpower production
being reduced. The overproduction of doctors has
led to current system changes, but on the other hand
created excessive demands for support. Government
policy making and health manpower training are
perhaps best characterised as the reactionary
'bounded rational' model described in Chapter 5.
    Employer policy makers appear to be a growing
influence in the United States and potentially could
have a great influence on health itself. Currently
many employers have reduced utilisation of health
services by adopting employee copayments thus
inserting financial barriers to care, apparently at
no sacrifice in health status. Other employers are
taking a more positive approach to reducing medical
care use by promoting health of employees and their
families through health education and self help

programmes. Increasing numbers of employers are
contracting for hospital claims review to evaluate
the quality as well as the quantity of care received
by their employees and families.

Legal System Influence

The legal system in the United States also
influences health service performance. Lawyers in
the United States may accept cases on the
contingency that the client pays only if the case is
won. Consequently paitents suspecting malpractice
have little to lose and possibly a great deal of
money to gain by suing doctors and hospitals. The
real threat of a malpractice suit is a powerful
financial incentive to practise high quality care.
On the other hand, it has also been a major
influence on rising costs of health care as doctors
have to practise defensively, ensuring that latest
technologies are used. Malpractice insurance is
also no small cost item for doctors, currently
around $8,000 annually for surgeons, but exceeding
$50,000 per year for some higher risk surgical
specialties in New York City. The importance of
malpractice litigation is likely to increase as PPS
and HMOs provide financial incentives for doctors to
do less medical service.

Management Influence

Health care managers are a growing force in
effective and efficient health service performance.
As noted previously, the recognition of hospital
administrators as chief executive officers and their
designation as 'president' is evidence of their
growing authority and accountability for
performance. Figure 8.1 portrayed differences in
efficiency and effectiveness among 13 acute
inpatient psychiatric units studied by Schulz,
Greenley, and Peterson (1983). They found that
managers of the more efficient (lower cost per
stay) and higher quality units had explicit goals
for efficiency and effectiveness, made more visible
the consequences of operation in terms of how the
unit was performing in relation to goals, and in
addition had more formal co-ordination policies,
more meetings and reports and more internal staff
education activities. There was also evidence that
higher quality but less efficient units managed
primarily for quality and mismanaged costs, and that
more efficient but lower quality units managed for

lower costs but mismanaged quality. The less
efficient and lower quality units were essentially
unmanaged. Managers of those units appeared to use
management practices as symbols, or ends in
themselves, rather than as means to achieve high
performance outcomes. Research from this and other
studies of management in a variety of industries
suggests it will be increasingly important for
health services managers to set goals for performance, make consequences of operation visible by
providing management information systems for feedback on success in achieving goals, and to be proactive in co-ordinating services to achieve goals.

Patient Influence

Finally, there is evidence in the United States that
patients will have an increasing role in determining
the efficiency and effectiveness of health services.
Patients have a role in complying with doctors'
recommendations for medications, exercise, diet, and
healthful behaviours such as avoiding tobacco. In
addition, patients in the United States are
beginning to take an active role in medical
decisions, asking for thorough explanations of
problems and treatment options, obtaining at least
second opinions from other doctors, and monitoring
their own medications and symptoms along with
doctors and nurses. A new and growing organisation
in the United States is the Peoples Medical Society
which helps consumers to select, monitor and
evaluate medical performace. HMOs and PPOs are
further developments which give consumers the
opportunity to evaluate and select efficient and
effective medical services through their purchasing
power. In the longer range it also appears that
self actuated care can be advanced through home
computers which might advance their own knowledge
for more effective and efficient health service and
their own optimum state of health.

In conclusion, health services in the United
States are currently undergoing changes which are
likely to continue progress towards efficiency and
effectiveness, and after some initial trauma more
acceptability in the longer term. Preliminary
evidence from Madison, Wisconsin, where current
changes appear to be more dramatic than elsewhere in
the United States, suggests there can be a fairly
compatible joint effort between providers, policy
makers, managers and consumers to implement changes
that will achieve higher performing systems.

Chapter 9

COMPARATIVE PERSPECTIVES ON PERFORMANCE

Andrew F. Long, Stephen Harrison, and
Geoffrey Mercer

The preceding theoretical and empirical Chapters of
this book have shown that the notion of health
services performance is complex and contentious,
resulting in variable policies over time and place.
In a 'rational' world there would be objectives or
standards to be met, arrangements for measuring the
match between actual events and the desired
standards, and a mechanism for correcting any
mismatch. (Dunsire 1978) This Chapter sets out to
compare and contrast the approaches adopted in the
studied countries (Chapters 6 to 8) with the
theoretical and conceptual indications outlined in
Chapters 1 to 5. Several aspects are discussed:
what are the origins of a concern with performance?
how is performance perceived and defined? and what
problems are faced in the implementation of
resulting policies? The Chapter concludes by
drawing attention to the implications of current
policies and in particular the neglect of
effectiveness, and argues for the pursuit of a more
extensive definition of performance.

ORIGINS OF A CONCERN WITH PERFORMANCE

In the three countries - Britain, Canada, and the
USA - public intervention in the funding and
regulation of health care has greatly expanded
during the post war period. It began earlier in
Britain with the inception of the NHS in 1947, but
significant growth was delayed for a decade in
Canada and the USA. Britain's NHS rested on a
general taxation based system, Canada pursued a
universal national health insurance scheme, while in
the USA a complex mixture of public and private
insurance schemes developed, and still exist, on a

categorical rather than universal basis (for example, Medicare and Medicaid). On the capital side, hospital construction and modernisation was emphasised in Canada (grants starting in the 1940s) and the USA (Hill Burton Act in 1946), with little at all in Britain until the Hospital Plan in the 1960s. Finally, medical education and research was actively encouraged in all three countries.

The growth and expansion up to the 1960s came under question with a declining world economy placing pressure on growth in the three countries. The extent and rising trend of government expenditure became a prime target for review. A gradual slowdown in hospital construction and in the provision of greater numbers of hospital acute beds per population occurred. At the same time, efforts to promote health, and a concern with the effects of lifestyle came to the fore with Lalonde (1974) in Canada, and with close parallels in the USA. In Britain, focus turned towards a more equitable means of allocating resources, and reorienting services towards nationally identified priority groups including prevention. (DHSS 1976c) Indeed, planning itself became a general catchword in the three countries, with a presumption that the expansion of health service costs would be controlled. In this way, the promotion of health services to meet health needs, on the developing lines of social equity, gave way to an emphasis on cost containment. Rising costs and attempts to control them thus became the spur and justification of interest in performance under the general heading of 'efficiency'.

PERCEPTIONS AND DEFINITIONS OF PERFORMANCE

The studies of Britain, Canada, and the USA therefore reveal three trends. Firstly, there was an expansion of health services (hospital based, and physician dominated) to promote access to high quality care. This growth was not in its early years subject to detailed or co-ordinated planning of resources or their allocation. Furthermore, effectiveness was not seen as an issue. Secondly, a turnaround in the expansionary policy occurred, first in Britain, then in North America. The last two decades have been marked by a developing concentration on cost-cutting and health planning exercises. Efficiency in the sense of containing costs become important with effectiveness raised as an adjunct to containment policies. There was further acknowledgement of the desirability of reallocating or redistributing resources, and differing mechanisms for its achievement. Thirdly, the 'medical model' came under increasing challenge. Attempts were made to bring medicine under closer control (though not to the same extent in Britain), as well as to develop alternative systems of delivery, and to encourage consumer involvement in health care, and health prevention. Against this background, how then was performance perceived and defined?

The varying perspectives of the different actors (funders, policy makers, health care practitioners and consumers) can be characterised in a general way for the three countries studied. Firstly, health care practitioners, especially the medical profession, have been generally concerned with maximising what Donabedian (1980) calls 'technical efficiency', that is the achievement of a customary protocol of diagnostic and treatment efforts which is held to maximise benefits to the patient. Operational objectives and priorities, as opposed to formal ones, have been set by the aggregate of decisions of individual physicians. A range of agencies with responsibility for monitoring aspects of performance have generally supported such definitions. For example, PROs in the USA and the Royal Colleges in Britain have in their different ways reinforced more intensive standards of treatment and diagnosis: PROs by reviewing the handling of actual cases and the Colleges by setting out minimum clinical facilities for the accreditation of training posts.

Pursuing Donabedian's (1980) differentiation between structure, process and outcome in quality assurance, all three countries have explored and pursued the structural aspect. In Britain, the emphasis has been on bureaucratic structural changes, ranging from the 1974 and 1982 reorganisations of the NHS, RAWP, and culminating in current developments surrounding the General Manager. In North America the concern has been more with the existence of facilities, their distribution and the role of outside agencies. Additionally, process has been reviewed in Canada and the USA through the role of the reimbursement system (PSROs, PROs and now DRGs). Current concerns in Britain with planning and performance review have recently turned attention onto process with limited success (Chapter 6). In none of the countries has outcome been a major thrust, notwithstanding the comments in Chapter 8 that there have been moves to health promotion, greater consumer participation in treatment choices, and resort to second opinions in the USA.

Secondly, in contrast with the practitioners, the funders (politicians and governments) have mainly focussed on distributive efficiency, or equity. Steps have been taken to provide health care for sections of the population who would otherwise not receive it: in the USA by targeting the elderly and the poor (through Medicare and Medicaid respectively) and in Canada by the provision of universal national health insurance. In Britain, with its existing open access to virtually free services, attention has been directed to the more equitable geographical allocation of resources, currently through the RAWP formula. It is thus noticeable that, notwithstanding free market rhetoric, in none of the countries has health care been left to market determination, though the size and role of the private sector varies considerably.

The stance of third-party payers for health care is more difficult to characterise. In Britain and Canada the payers are governments, who in both cases have succeeded in restricting health care expenditure. In the USA, insurers have experimented with various devices for controlling and reducing costs (such as mandatory second opinions concerning surgery), but major attention has only really emanated from the effect of rising premia upon employers' payroll costs.

Thirdly, the performance orientations of consumers seem to have been largely aligned with those of health practitioners, as was graphically portrayed in Chapter 4. Technical quality of care is the keystone, but country differences are easily apparent. In the USA the physician-patient relationship is premised on the assumption of a 'right to know' for the consumer and thus to make an informed judgement about allowing a treatment to commence, whilst in Britain the patient plays a more passive role. Again the Canadian experience would seem to lie in between. In addition, the very culture surrounding medical practice differs. Klein (1984 p. 144) reviewing Aaron and Schwartz (1984) comments on the 'humane clinical conservatism in Britain' and 'the heroic aggressive style of medicine in the USA', and the very perceptions of illness and debility as 'the natural order of things' (in Britain) with consequential deferential patients in contrast to 'the perfectability of man' (in the USA) with illness seen as a challenge to action, and patients as a result becoming demanding consumers. Such cultures, he argues, help to explain and compound the differing rates of expenditure in the two countries. Illich's (1976) comments on social iatrogenesis are also relevant here.

As governments have recently become concerned with the costs of health care, so too have practitioners started to accede to this. Challenges to clinical freedom are becoming more widely voiced, along with various forms of clinical budgetting, whilst in the USA health maintenance organisations have given substance to such concerns. It is important to note that in all three countries the basis of this attention is much more with total costs than with the particular aspects of efficiency elucidated in Chapter 3.

This recent focus on cost control has been shrouded in rhetoric. If a government wishes to maintain simultaneous concerns with overall costs and the avoidance of additional inequities, it cannot be declared that reduced inputs will result in service deterioration. It is however equally interesting to ask why funders and policy makers have not until recently attempted to impose their view of performance on health practitioners. Only to a limited extent can this be understood through literature on external control (Chapter 5). For the health care agencies in all three countries have been for some time considerably dependent upon government resources. One development is the increased willingness of governments to use the potential power which they possess: a pushing to one side of the intermediate monitoring agencies and the substitution of direct government involvement.

Perhaps, given the growing workload of governments, this involvement is something of a blunt instrument. The potentially more subtle instruments of planning and policy guidelines have been denigrated in order to save money. Hence, it is not surprising that policies have perverse consequences. In Britain, it is likely that cuts in resources will chiefly affect the care groups (such as the elderly) which are the official priorities, whilst in the USA the operation of DRGs seems likely to affect prestigious tertiary institutions more than others. If the overriding aim is to save money, then these distributional issues are of little real concern to governments. The relative power of the affected groups may however result in a

modification of policies: for the elderly little
improvement, while for prestigious medical
institutions, a more optimistic prospect.

It is also possible to conclude that health
practitioners are able to sidestep initial cost-
cutting exercises. For the burden of initial
manpower lay-offs have largely fallen on hospital
workers not involved in direct patient care, with
much criticism in Britain, for example, of the
'administrative tail'. As noted in Chapter 5, such
categories of worker are easy targets as
scapegoats.

In conclusion, two points must be noted.
Firstly, all the operational definitions which have
been discussed are consonant with the 'medical
model' of health and illness identified in Chapter
2. Secondly, and simultaneously, all manage to
ignore the effectiveness considerations discussed in
the same Chapter. Only insofar as health
practitioners give attention to the technical aspect
of the quality of care is it addressed. Health
outcomes are little explored, as is the relative
role of health services in bringing about changes in
health status.

PROBLEMS IN POLICY IMPLEMENTATION

Given the varying perceptions and definitions of
performance of the participants in health care
delivery, planning and policy making it is not
surprising that problems in implementing policies
aimed at monitoring and improving performance have
arisen. Firstly, there are genuine problems in
defining objectives and devising relevant
information systems. Performance definitions are
contentious partly (though, as argued above, not
only) because notions of health status and health
service effectiveness are complex and sometimes
obscure. Indeed, performance has been evaluated
according to organisational objectives, whereas
bounded rational theories predict it is unlikely
that any of the main organisational actors involved
(except for consumers) have much interest or
inclination to take a broader perspective.

Secondly, government behaviour in all three
countries seems essentially reactive rather than
proactive. Reaction to a perceived economic crisis
has led to a changed priority from equity to overall
costs, a solution to which perhaps conservative
governments are ideologically predisposed.

Thirdly, it is therefore not surprising that relevant information on health services performance has been rejected or ignored. In Britain, the relative cheapness of the NHS by international comparison has not altered the perception that it is too expensive; nor have the recommendations of the Black Report (Townsend and Davidson 1982) for reducing inequalities in health been taken up (an interest in relative effectiveness or allocative efficiency). A similar scenario exists in North America.

Fourthly, there are suggestions of poorly thought through cause-effect relationships. For example, Neuhauser (1983) has shown some of the unintended consequences inherent in the DRG system, and Barnard and Harrison (1984) have argued that the implementation of the Griffiths Report, that is, the appointment of General Managers in place of consensus teams, risks weakening management rather than strengthening it. However, it would appear that attempts to monitor innovations such as HMOs in the USA have been more thorough than British attempts.

Fifthly, there is the question of how actors succeed in imposing policies upon others. It is clear that governments through their provision of financial resources to health services have considerable power. However, until recently it has been possible for health care practitioners and institutions to avoid being subject to this: that is, whilst ever government concerns have been with health care needs. Health practitioners have not surprisingly been able to claim special authority over the interpretation. Thus, in Britain, government health care priorities have made little advance, as Chapter 6 shows graphically. More recently governments have tried to contain and save expenditure, a fairly specific priority not subject to practitioners' interpretation, except insofar as it has enforced rationing decisions on health care. What seems to be the case is that the public control of the health sector's resources has had a global rather than a specific orientation. Governments can cut spending, but find it difficult to indicate just where this cut should occur, the latter question being subject to health practitioners' (and potentially consumers') interpretations. This is perhaps advantageous to governments since it decentralises blame, and the difficult ethical decisions over who should get what and how much care.

Furthermore, there is the suggestion that the applicability of management techniques is doomed to no better than partial success because they simply cut right across the organisation of medical practice. Effective regulation of professional activities is difficult because of the extent of medical power. It would also be misplaced, because it has only provided mechanisms for enhancing the organisational efficiency of the health institutions as opposed to the health status of the population. Until there is some agreement on what acceptable outputs of health care are, and how they can be measured, managerialism will not make a positive impression. It is equally problematic because of the confusion created by the observation that completely different systems of health care come up with rather similar results.

In addition, policy on structural interests in health care, and their battle for policy making control amplifies the political problems in implementing health planning. For example, Alford (1975) highlights the particular conflict between the dominant 'professional monopolists' and the challenges from the 'corporate rationalisers'. Klein (1983), on the NHS, talks about 'veto power' and 'corporate stalemate'. This points to the confusion and complexities of health planning and policy making: of dynamics without change. Others have extended this argument and suggested that there are structural constraints in a capitalist society on state intervention in health services, in particular an inability to overturn the fact that capitalism is 'bad for your health'. Questions are then raised about the range of factors seen as causes of illness, and also the potential contribution of health services to health.

In conclusion, problems of implementation are legion, ranging from ambiguity in policy aims and responsibilities, the problems of relating general guidance (for example on priorities) to particular cases, enforcment, changing financial and manpower assumptions or conditions, and differing time horizons of actors (the planners versus the health practitioners), and organisational and political factors. Furthermore, if actors in health services do not agree over what is meant by 'performance' and would not in any event know how to achieve it, the results of their interactions are largely indeterminate. As Thompson and Tuden (1956) observed, where there is agreement about neither means nor ends, then the only basis of decision is 'inspiration'!

IMPLICATIONS OF CURRENT POLICIES AND POTENTIAL DEVELOPMENTS

The review of current approaches and perceptions of health services performance, and their implications, in the USA, Canada, and Britain has highlighted the overriding current importance of efficiency or, more specifically, of cost containment. Such a comment applies at a general macro level, within a (micro) clinical setting of attempts to provide high (technical) quality of care to patients, albeit in the context of rationing. The overall thrust of performance and health service evaluation, with its three interdependent components of effectiveness, efficiency, and acceptability, has thus been narrowly perceived, defined and implemented.

Indeed, the apparent failure of efficiency, or rather cost containment exercises, has promoted interest in the re-privatisation of health services based on suggestions that there exist fundamental institutional barriers to promoting efficiency in a publicly funded and regulated system. Thus efficiency is reinterpreted to downgrade any notion of equity; that is, it is based on restricting access on a universal basis, or greatly restricting the range of services which would be so covered. Increasing competition between public and private modes is sought, especially in the USA. In Britain and Canada re-privatisation concentrates on user charges and a greater element of private medical practice. There is too an increasing confrontation between the medical profession and governments over the payment of physicians. In the USA this has meant expansion of PROs and certificate of need, and in Canada fights over extra-billing and fee-schedules.

It is also evident that the expansion of health services has provided the imbalance which current containment policies are seeking to overcome. The implementation of health planning exercises to rationalise, to regionalise, to cut costs, and to promote health, have been singularly less successful. Even so, equity through expansion has not greatly reduced the differences in health status, as opposed to the formal access to health care. Efforts to reallocate services on a more equitable basis in a time of general cost containment seem largely to have been thwarted. In

Canada, perhaps, the problem is less because priority areas were not formulated with the same precision as in Britain; and in the USA yet another form of decentralised health planning has equally failed to control costs or to reallocate resources. Indeed, the plethora of HSAs, PROs, HMOs, and even DRGs has yet failed to severely dent the USA's position as the biggest per capita health spender of the three countries. One could speculate here on the effect of the USA pursuing a policy of universal health insurance on Canadian lines. It would certainly be in a better position to contain costs judging by the present Canadian experience. Equity would also be improved, and in this way the impact of the health care system.

A major question which must at least be addressed is that of why efficiency, or more particularly cost containment under the label of managerial efficiency, has been the focus of attention rather than any of the other aspects of efficiency or performance in general. Indeed, there is an explicit neglect of a stated concern with the effectiveness of health services, a priori the most fundamental and critical area in any performance evaluation. Several comments can be made. Firstly, effectiveness in terms of beneficial effects on individual patients' health, and the more general issue of the impact of health services, is a difficult phenomenon to assess: what criteria should be used, whether assessment should be made of long or short term benefits, and so on. Moreover, it is not an area of immediate interest to funders and policy makers. Their concern lies more with the use and control of resources. Efficiency, in fact both managerial and distributive, is thus their forte. As Vuori (1982) argues, effectiveness is a key issue for the consumer and also the health practitioner in their face-to-face contacts. Secondly, efficiency in its managerial sense is an easier concept to handle. Thirdly, in terms of Donabedian's (1980) three components of quality assurance, the consumer is almost by definition concerned with outcome, while the funders' and policy makers' interests are likely to reside in structure and process. Fourthly, where the funders have to become involved in an interest in outcome in the broader political arena, the debate tends to be carried out at the level of, for example, changes in life expectancy, increases in longevity, or changes in perinatal mortality rates with little concern for issues of cause and effect, or the relative contribution of health services to these changes. Klein's (1982) comments are of obvious relevance; performance does indeed depend on one's location in the health care system.

In this way, the funders and policy makers seem to be concerned with effectiveness in the more general sense of the achievement of organisational objectives. For example, whether the health services meet their targets on cash limits and budgets or manpower ceilings, or crude indicators of input and activity, become the main areas of interest, satisfying the more general political and ideological context in which performance and evaluation is based: in Britain Parliament, DHSS and health authorities; in the USA insurance companies and the federal government through the use of, for example, DRGs; and in Canada similar budgetting limits in federal and provincial arrangements. So, 'organisational effectiveness' and not the potential impact of health services on the population becomes the aim.

The health practitioner too is not necessarily overly concerned with health status changes. The relevant notion is rather that of the quality of care (technical efficiency): that is, meeting professionally determined and acceptable (acknowledged) standards of care. The implication is that such a standard of care is effective in the sense of a beneficial effect on health status. But, as has been pointed out in Chapter 2, many treatments are unevaluated. Further, when challenged regarding effectiveness the notion of clinical freedom may be raised. The dominance of the medical model of what constitutes illness, the causes of illness and appropriate forms of intervention, treatment, care and cure, and the power of the medical profession become critical items to take into account.

It is then perhaps unsurprising that effectiveness is not pursued within the context of performance given its lack of interest and political relevance to the funders and policy makers, and its potential threat to the power base of the major group of health practitioners, the physicians. Further, there is no incentive for local level managers to explore effectiveness if it is not a valued goal. The concern with managerial efficiency and the achievement of organisational objectives is sufficient and makes political sense.

However, the pursuit of efficiency, or rather strict cost control, is also unattractive from the health practitioner's perspective. Underfunding becomes the physician's cry while the policy makers perceive overfunding. Cost controls threaten to break into the area of clinical freedom, and also place the health practitioner in the role of enforcing explicit rationing of health services. Available finance is not sufficient to meet demand. At least in the British context, this is managed in an apparently satisfactory manner by health practitioners pointing to the lack of funds as the cause of rationing; in other circumstances the patient would receive treatment. Further, in both Britain and Canada, resort to private medicine can be made, with consequent financial gain for those involved. In the USA, Aaron and Schwartz (1984) point to the possibility of litigation and use of the Canadian system, once (and if) such rationing due to cost containment becomes a reality. Exactly how the courts will respond is unknown. The issue resolves around the denial of a potentially beneficial therapy. Aaron and Schwartz foresee the situation of a gradual redefinition of negligence, moving in line with the courts' present reference to 'customary standards of medical practice'.

So far, possible reasons for a sole focus of attention on managerial efficiency and to the disregard of other aspects of efficiency and effectiveness have been outlined. What of acceptability? The professional's viewpoint has been discussed already. Where this leaves the consumer is doubtful; resort to the use of political power (in elections and through pressure groups) and to the courts appears to be the only option. Even then, effectiveness may not be assessed, at least on the experience of litigation in the USA with its reference to normal professional standards. Equity of access and technical efficiency alone may be pursued.

A comparison with private industry is perhaps apposite. There, product quality is continually assessed. Technical efficiency, managerial efficiency and the achievement of organisational objectives are key goals. As for acceptability, advertising either attempts to manipulate consumer demand or supports and feeds on an already existing need for the product. The analogy to health services is close. In neither can one argue that consumers' own needs, as self-perceived, are addressed. The health professionals define needs and structure appropriate responses to them. In addition, consumers have expectations of health services. But how are such expectations built up? As Illich (1976) comments, social and structural iatrogenesis has arisen. The consumers' dependence on the health practitioners is manipulated and expanded against their own wider inderests.

The outlook does then look bleak for the adoption of a more extensive perception, definition, approach and pursuit of health services performance. However, the current approach of managerial efficiency and services at minimum cost, without any apparent concern with their effectiveness and acceptability, is not without its critics, as Chapter 6 indicated. A change in emphasis from cost containment to effectiveness, acceptability and efficiency can, it would seem, only come from a changed political commitment to health services evaluation itself, irrespective of any of the practical difficulties of objective setting, measurement, information, and acting on identified mismatches, with all this entails for the organisational actors' interests (Chapter 5).

One possible line of development is for services, both current and any proposed developments and modifications, to be reviewed according to criteria such as those indicated in the review checklist in Table 2.3 , with the addition of questions on acceptability. That is, any request would have to be justified in terms of its need, expected outcome, impact on the community's state of health, acceptability (to consumers and health practitioners), and cost grounds. In McCarthy's (1982) terms, epidemiolgocal targets should be set. Taking this a stage further, any resource used by a departmental manager would then be monitored in line with clearly stated objectives (in terms of effects on patients' health status), and decisions taken to increase their achievements. Such a process could be applied to clinical practice itself; for example, routine surgery might be undertaken first with a beneficial effect on waiting lists (maximising impact), and then the more specialised where fewer benefit. Ethical issues clearly arise.

Such an approach is however premised on a rational comprehensive model of decision making and organisational behaviour. Following the logic of Chapter 3, decisions about objectives would have to be made, and much more (and detailed) information about marginal costs and benefits obtained. If actors did not agree about these matters, then ways would have to be sought to impose one actor's (for example, the general manager's) definition on the rest. An alternative would be the adoption of an incremental approach, where actors dissatisfied with the present state of affairs construct <u>ad hoc</u> strategies aimed at improving the situation. Further if a more extensive definition of performance, building on the discussions in Chapters 2, 3, and 4, is to be imposed then far more sophisticated systems of incentives and control will have to be devised than has hitherto been the case.

Any such initiatives have though to occur within a context of medically dominated health services, and in particular a narrow view of the causes of illness, playing down the role of structural economic and political features of society, and a limited consideration of the relevance to health status of factors outside the health services. Indeed, if one considers the situation of health status in Britain, would an injection of more funds into the NHS result in larger gains in general health and welfare than their injection into aspects of the socio-economic environment, such as housing and employment? And if such money were added to the NHS, would it go into health promotion, where longer as opposed to shorter term benefits would be anticipated? While peer review may be an acceptable and effective way of reviewing professional provision of care (that is, in terms of its achievement of customary standards), it alone is unlikely to contribute to a shift in emphasis to outcome and effectiveness in general. Finally, one can ask how additional funds would be spent if given to doctors to spend as they deem fit. Would those with greatest power gain most, or would rational priorities based on the community's health needs dominate the allocative procedure?

The prevailing emphasis on cost containment will indeed cut out 'waste' from health service systems (a desirable aim), but there is no guarantee that it will either eradicate all waste, or leave 'useful' (that is, effective and acceptable) services untouched. As Maxwell and his colleagues (1983) have argued, a broader concern than managerial efficiency must be pursued, requiring balance with an equal concern with quality. '... Indicators of impact, satisfaction, and (in a negative sense) the absence of avoidable errors' (p. 48) need to be developed and employed as tools in performance review. The pursuit of waste, itself an imprecise notion, can only lead to further dilemmas about rationing health care, and consequent unpopularity on the part of consumers and health practitioners.

Health services, with their connotations of the 'deserving poor' and the recognition that illness is a risk all face and will one day succumb to, remain a uniquely popular segment of public welfare provision. The erosion of provision compared with expectations cannot continue indefinitely. Exploring the effectiveness, efficiency and acceptability of service provision, while itself not unproblematic, at least shifts attention to key issues, which have as an expected outcome an increase in the health status of the population at large, surely the desideratum of health services.

BIBLIOGRAPHY

Aaron, H.J. and Schwartz, W.B. (1984) The Painful
    Prescription: Rationing Hospital Care,
    Brookings Institution, Washington D.C.
Abel-Smith, B. and Titmuss, R. (1956) The Cost of
    the National Health Service in England and
    Wales, Cambridge University Press, Cambridge
Alderson, M. (ed) (1982) The Prevention of Cancer,
    Edward Arnold (Publishers) Ltd., London
Alford, R. (1975) Health Care Politics, University
    of Chicago Press, Chicago
Allen, D.E. (1979) Hospital Planning: The
    Development of the 1962 Hospital Plan, Pitman
    Medical, Tunbridge Wells
Allen, D.E. (1983) 'The Relationship Between the
    DHSS and Health Authorities' in D.E. Allen and
    J.A. Hughes (eds.), Management for Health
    Authorities, Pitman, London
Allison, G.T. (1969) 'Conceptual Models and the
    Cuban Missile Crisis', American Political
    Science Review, vol.. LXIII no. 3, September
Altman, S. and Blendon, R. (1979) (eds) Medical
    Technology: The Culprit Behind Health Care
    Costs?, US Government Printing Office,
    Washington DC
Andreopoulos, S. (1975) (ed.) National Health
    Insurance: Can We Learn From Canada?, Wiley,
    Toronto
Anthony, R. and Herzlinger, R. (1975) Management
    Control in Non-Profit Organisations, Irwin
    Homewood
Antonovsky, A. (1973) 'The Utility of the Breakdown
    Concept', Social Science and Medicine, vol.
    7, pp. 605-12
Antonovsky, A. (1980) Health Stress and Coping (New
    Perspectives on Mental and Physical Well-
    Being), Jossey-Bass Publications, London

Bibliography

Association of Medical Records Officers (1983)
   'Measuring the Quality', Health and Social
   Services Journal, 1 December, p. 144
Aucoin, P. (1974) 'Federal Health Care Policy' in
   G.B. Doern and V.S. Wilson (eds) Issues in
   Canadian Public Policy, Macmillan, Toronto,
   pp. 55-84
Austin, C.J. (1979) Information Systems for Hospital
   Administration, Health Administration Press,
   Ann Arbor
Babson, J.H. (1973) Disease Costing, Manchester
   University Press, Manchester
Bachrach, P. and Baratz, M.S. (1970) Power and
   Poverty, Oxford University Press, London
Badgley, R. and Smith, D.A. (1979) User Charges for
   Health Services, Ontario Council of Health
Bailey, N.J.T. (1975) 'System Modelling in Health
   Planning' in N.J.T. Bailey and M. Thompson
   (eds), System Aspects of Health Planning,
   North-Holland, New York
Bakke, E.W. (1959) 'Concepts of Social Organisations
   in Modern Organisation Theory' in M. Haire
   (ed.), Modern Organisation Theory, John Wiley,
   New York
Banks, G.T. (1979) 'Programme Budgetting in the NHS'
   in T.T Booth (ed.) Planning for Welfare: Social
   Policy and the Expenditure Process, Basil
   Blackwell and Martin Robertson, Oxford
Barer, M.L., Evans, R.G. and Stoddart, G.L. (1979)
   Controlling Health Care Costs by Direct Charges
   to Patients: Snare or Delusion?, Occasional
   Paper no. 10, Ontario Economic Council,
   Toronto
Barnard, K. and Harrison, S. (1984) 'Memorandum on
   the Griffiths Report', First Report from the
   Social Services Committee for the Session 1983-
   84, House of Commons Paper no. 209, HMSO,
   London
Barnes, K.S. (1984) 'Health Authority Performance
   Indicators', Hospital and Health Services
   Review, May, pp. 118-119
Beck, R.G. (1973) 'Economic Class and Access to
   Physician Services under Public Medical Care
   Insurance', International Journal of Health
   Services, 3, 3, p. 341-55
Beer, S.H. (1981) Brain of the Firm: The Managerial
   Cybernetics of Organisation, John Wiley,
   Chichester

Bibliography

Bernard, C. (1927) An Introduction to the Study of Experimental Medicine, English Translation, Greene, H.C., Schuman, New York (reprinted 1949)

Bevan, R.G. and Spencer, A.H. (1984) 'Models of Resources Policy of Regional Health Authorities' in M. Clarke (ed.) Planning and Analysis in Health Care Systems, Pion, London

Bierman, H. and Schmidt, S. (1980) The Capital Budgetting Decision: Economic Analysis of Investment Projects, Collier-Macmillan, New York, 5th Edition

Black, E., Cooper, J., and Landry, G. (1978) Health Care in Manitoba, Canadian Union of Public Employees, Winnipeg, Manitoba

Blau, P.M. (1955) The Dynamics of Bureaucracy, University of Chicago Press, Chicago

Blishen, B.R. (1964) Doctors and Doctrines: The Ideology of Medical Care in Canada, University of Toronto Press, Toronto

Breslow, L. (1972) 'A Quantitative Approach to the World Health Organisation Definition of Health: Physical, Mental and Social Well-Being', International Journal of Epidemiology, vol. 1, pp. 347-55

Brewster, C.J., Gill, C.G., and Richbell, S. (1981) 'Developing an Analytical Approach to Industrial Relations Policy', Personnel Review 10 (2)

British Columbia (1973) Health Security for British Columbians, Foulkes Report, Province of British Columia, Victoria

Brook, R.H. and Appel, F.A. (1973) 'Quality of Care Assessment: Choosing a Method for Peer Review', New England Journal of Medicine, 288: 25, pp. 1323-1329, June 21

Brooks, R. (1984) Financial Information Systems in the NHS, Paper presented to Institute of Cost and Management Accountants Conference, 1 May

Bross, I.D.J. (1981) Scientific Strategies to Save Your Life: A Statistical Approach to Primary Prevention, Marcel Dekker Inc., New York

Brown, R.G.S. (1975) The Management of Welfare, Fontana, London

Buckley, M.H., Buckley, J.W. and Plank, T.M. (1980) SEC Accounting, John Wiley, New York

Buxton, M.J. and West, R.R. (1975) 'Cost-Benefit Analysis of Long-Term Haemodialysis for Chronic Renal Failure', British Medical Journal, 17 May

Campbell, D.T. (1969) 'Reforms as Experiments', American Psychologist, vol. 24, pp. 409-29; reprinted in Bynner, J. and Stribley, K.M. (eds) (1979) Social Research: Principles and Procedures, Longman, London, pp. 79-112

Canada (1964-5) Report, Royal Commission on Health Services, Queen's Printer, Ottawa

Canada, Department of Health and Welfare (1970) Report of the Task Force on the Cost of the Health Services, Information Canada, Ottawa

Canada, Department of Health and Welfare (1972) The Community Health Centre in Canada, Information Canada, Ottawa

Canada, Department of Health and Welfare (1974) A New Perspective on the Health of Canadains: A Working Document, (Lalonde Report), Information Canada, Ottawa

Canada, Department of Health and Welfare (1980) Canada's National-Provincial Health Programs for the 1980s, (Hall Report), Information Canada, Ottawa

Canada, Department of Health and Welfare (1983a) National Health Expenditures in Canada 1979-1982, Department of Health and Welfare, Ottawa

Canada, Department of Health and Welfare (1983b) Preserving Universal Medicare, Queen's Printer, Ottawa

Canada, House of Commons (1981) Report of the Parliamentary Task Force: Fiscal Federalism in Canada, Information Canada, Ottawa

Canada, House of Commons, (1984) Minutes of Proceedings and Evidence of the Standing Committee on Health, Welfare and Social Affairs, Second Session of 32nd Parliament, Issues 1-18, Queen's Printer, Ottawa

Canadian Medical Association (1981) Submission to Parliamentary Task Force on Federal-Provincial Fiscal Arrangements, Canadian Medical Association, Ottawa

Canadian Medical Association (1984a) Submission to the House of Commons Standing Committee on Health, Welfare and Social Affairs, re: Bill C3, Canadian Medical Association, Ottawa

Canadian Medical Assocation (1984b) Submission to the Task Force on the Allocation of Health Care Resources, Canadian Medical Association, Ottawa

Carlson, R.J. (1975) The End of Medicine, John Wiley, New York

Carter, C.O. and Peel, J. (1976) (ed.) Equalities and Inequalities in Health, Academic Press, London

Champagne, F., Contandriopoulos, A-P., Fornier, M-A. and Laurier, C. (1983) 'Pursuit of Equity, Respect of Liberties and Control of Health Care Costs in Quebec', unpublished paper, University of Montreal

Charles, C. (1976) 'The Medical Profession and Health Insurance: An Ontario Case Study', Social Science and Medicine, 10, pp. 33-8

Charlton, J.R.H., Silver, R., Hartley, R.M., and Holland, W.W. (1983) 'Geographical Variations in Mortality from Conditions Amenable to Medical Intervention in England and Wales', The Lancet, March 25

Child, J. (1977) Organisation: A Guide to Problems and Practice, Harper and Row

Clarke, K. (1984), quoted in 'Clarke Welcomes Oxford's Aims', Hospital and Health News of Appointments Review, May 30

Clayden, A.D. (1984) 'Training Decision Makers to Plan', Paper presented to the 10th Annual Conference of the European Working Group on Operational Research Applied to Health Services, Venice, June

Clute, K.F. (1963) The General Practitioner: A Study of Medical Education and Practice in Ontario and Nova Scotia, University of Toronto Press, Toronto

Coburn, D., D'Arcy, C., New, P. and Torrance, G. (eds) (1981) Health and Canadian Society: Sociological Perspectives, Fitzhenry and Whiteside, Toronto

Coburn, D., Torrance, G. and Kauvert, J. (1983) 'Medical Dominance in Canada in Historical Perspective', International Journal of Health Services, 13, 3, pp. 407-32

Cochrane, A.L. (1972) Effectiveness and Efficiency: Random Reflections on Health Services, Nuffield Provincial Hospitals Trust, London

Colby, D.E. and Begley, C.E. (1983) 'The Effects of Implementation Problems on Certificate of Need Decisions in Illinois', Health Policy and Education, vol. 13 no. 4, April

Collins Dictionary of the English Language (1980), Collins, London and Glasgow

Collville, I. (1982) Accounting Information Systems in a Police Force, Research Paper, University of Bath

Bibliography

Cook   T.D. and Reichard, T.C.S. (eds) (1979)
    Qualitative   and   Quantitative   Methods in
    Evaluation Research,   Sage   University
    Publications, New York
Cook,   T.D. and Campbell, D.T. (1979) Quasi-
    Experimentation Design and Analysis Issues for
    Field Settings, Rand McNally College Publishing
    Company, Chicago
Cooper, W. (1966) The Prices and Profits in the
    Pharmaceutical   Industry,   Pergamon   Press,
    Oxford
Cousins,   N.   (1979)   Anatomy of an Illness as
    Perceived by the Patient, W.W. Norton, New
    York
Cousins, N. (1983) The Healing Heart, W.W. Norton,
    New York
Craig,   J. (1983) 'The Growth of the Elderly
    Population', Population Trends no. 32 Summer,
    Office of Population Censuses and Surveys,
    HMSO, London, pp. 28-33
Crichton, A. (1976) 'The Shift from Entrepreneurial
    to Political Power in the Canadian Health
    System', Social Science and Medicine, 10, pp.
    59-66
Crichton, A. (1984) 'The Canadian Health Services
    System' in C.). Pannenborg, van der Werff, A.
    Hirsch, G.B. and Barnard, K. (eds) Reorienting
    Health Services, Plenum Press, London
Crossman,   R.H.S. (1972) A Politician's View of
    Health Service Planning, University of Glasgow
    Press, Glasgow
Crozier, M. (1964) The Bureaucratic Phenomenon,
    University of Chicago Press, Chicago
Culvez, A. and Blanchet, M. (1983) 'Potential Gains
    in Life Expectancy Free of Disability: A Tool
    For Health Planning', International Journal of
    Epidemiology, vol. 12, no 2, pp. 224-9
Cyert, R.M. and March, J.G. (1963) A Behavioural
    Theory of the Firm, Prentice-Hall, Englewood
    Cliffs NJ
DHSS   (1972) 'Management Arrangements for the
    Reorganised National Health Service, HMSO,
    London
DHSS   (1974) Democracy in the National Health
    Service, HMSO, London
DHSS (1976a) The NHS Planning System, DHSS, London
DHSS (1976b) Priorities for Health and Personal
    Social Services, HMSO, London
DHSS   (1976c)   Sharing Resources for Health in
    England, The Report of the Resource Allocation
    Working Party, HMSO, London

Bibliography

DHSS (1977) The Way Forward, HMSO, London
DHSS (1979) Patients First, HMSO, London
DHSS (1981a) Report of a Study on the Respective Roles of the General Acute and Geriatric Sectors in Care of the Elderly Hospital Patient, HMSO, London
DHSS (1981b) Care in Action: A Handbook of Policies and Priorities for the Health and Personal Social Services in England, Her Majesty's Stationery Office, London
DHSS (1982) Health Services Development: The NHS Planning System, HC(82)6, DHSS, London
DHSS (1983) NHS Management Inquiry Report, 'Griffiths Report', London
DHSS (1984) Health Services Development Resource Distribution for 1984-85, Services Priorities, Manpower and Planning, HC(84)2/LAC(84)4, January
Dahl, R.A. (1963) Modern Political Analysis, Prentice-Hall, Englewood Cliffs
Dingwall, R. (1976) Aspects of Illness, Martin Robertson, London
Doll, R. (1974) 'Survellance and Monitoring', International Journal of Epidemiology, vol. 3, no 4, pp. 305-14
Doll, R., and Peto, R. (1981) The Causes of Cancer, Oxford University Press, Oxford
Donabedian, A. (1980) The Definition of Quality and Approached to the Assessment, (volume 1 of Explorations in Quality Assessment and Monitoring), Health Administration Press, Michigan
Donabedian, A. (1966) 'Evaluating the Quality of Medical Care', Milbank Memorial Fund Quarterly vol. 64, no. 3, part 2, pp. 166-206
Downey, G. (1983) 'How Efficient is the NHS?', Hospital and Services Review, May, pp. 117-121
Doyal, L. and Epstein, S.S. (1983) Cancer in Britain: The Politics of Prevention, Pluto Press, London
Doyal, L. (1979) The Political Economy of Health, Pluto Press, London
Drucker, P. (1979) Management, Pan Books, London
Drummond, M.F. (1980) Principles of Economic Appraisal in Health Care, Oxford University Press, London
Duffee, D.E., and Klofas, J. (1983) 'Organisational Mandates and Client Careers: An Examination of Penal Policy', in Hall and Quinn (eds.), Organisational Theory (q.v.)

Dunsire, A. (1978) Implementation in a Bureaucracy, Martin Robertson and Oxford University Press, London

Eakin, J.M. (1984) 'Hospital Power Structure and the Democratisation of Hospital Administration in Quebec', Social Science and Medicine, vol. 18, no. 3, pp. 221-228

Enthoven, A.C. (1978) 'Consumer-Choice Health Plan: Inflation and Inequity in Health Care Today: Alternatives for Cost Control and an Analysis of Proposals for National Health Insurance', New England Journal of Medicine, 298: 650-658, March 23

Evans, R.G. (1982a) 'Health Care Funding in Canada: Patterns in Funding and Regulation' in G. McLachlan and A. Maynard (eds) The Public/Private Mix for Health, Nuffield Provincial Hospitals Trust, London.

Evans, R.G. (1982b) 'The Fiscal Management of Medical Technology: the case of Canada' in H.D. Banta (ed.) Resources for Health, Praeger, New York, pp. 178-199

Evans, R.G. (1982c) 'A Retrospective on the New Perspective', Journal of Health Politics, Policy and Law, 7, 2, pp. 325-44

Evans, R.G. (1983) 'Health Care in Canada: Patterns of Funding and Regulation', Journal of Health Policy and Law, 8, 1, pp. 1-43

Fairey, M.J. (1983) 'The Korner Report and its Implementation', Hospital and Health Services Review, July, pp. 180-182

Fanshel, S. (1972) 'A Meaningful Measure of Health for Epidemiology', International Journal of Epidemiology, vol. 1, pp. 319-37

Fayol, H. (1971) 'General Industrial Management', reprinted in D.S. Pugh (ed.), Organisational Theory, Penguin Books, Harmondsworth

Fishkin, J.S. (1979) Tyranny and Legitimacy: A Critique of Political Theories, Johns Hopkins University Press, Baltimore

Flexner, A. (1910) Medical Education in the United States and Canada, Carnegie Foundation for the Advancement of Teaching (reprinted by Science and Health Publications, Washington D.C.

Fowler, N. (1983) 'Statement on National Health Service Management Inquiry', House of Commons, 25 October

Fox, A. (1966) Industrial Sociology and Industrial Relations, HMSO, London

Bibliography

Freeborn, D.K. and Greenlick, M.R. (1973) 'Evaluation of the Performance of Ambulatory Care Systems: Research Requirements and Opportunities', Supplement to Medical Care, vol. 11, pp. 68-75

Freidson, E. (1970) Profession of Medicine: A Study of the Sociology of Applied Knowledge, Dodd Mean and Company, New York

Friedman, M. (1980) Free to Choose: A Personal Statement, Secker and Warburg, London

Galbraith, J.K. (1963) American Capitalism: The Concept of Countervailing Power, Pelican, Harmondsworth

Ghana Health Assessment Project Team (1981) 'A Quantitative Method for Assessing the Health Impact of Different Diseases in Less Developed Countries', International Journal of Epidemiology, vol. 10, no 1, pp. 73-80

Glaser, B.G. and Strauss, A.L. (1968) The Discovery of Grounded Theory: Strategies for Qualitative Research, Weidenfeld and Nicholson, London

Glennerster, H. (1983) Planning for Priority Groups, Martin Robertson, Oxford

Godbout, J. (1981) 'Is Consumer Control Possible in Health Care Services? The Quebec Case', International Journal of Health Services, 11, 1, pp. 151-67

Goldsmith, S. (1984) Theory 'Z' Hospital Management, Aspen Books, New York

Gosselin, R. (1984) 'Decentralisation/ Regionalisation: The Quebec Experience', Health Care Management Review, 9, 1, pp. 7-25

Gray, J.A.M. (1983) 'Four Box Model of Health Care: Development in a Time of Zero Growth', The Lancet, 19 November, pp. 1185-6

Grove, J.W. (1969) Organised Medicine in Ontario, Queen's Printer, Toronto

Gunn, L.A. (1978) 'Why is Implementation so Difficult?', Management Services in Government, vol. 33, no. 4, November

Hagard, S. Carter, F. and Milne, R.G. (1976) 'Screening for Spina Bifida Cystica: a Cost-Benefit Analysis', British Journal of Preventive and Social Medicine, vol. 30, pp. 40-53

Hall, R.H. and Quinn, R.L. (1983) (eds) Organisational Theory and Public Policy, Sage, Beverly Hills, California

Hallas, J. (1976) CHCs in Action, Nuffield Provincial Hospitals Trust, London

Bibliography

Ham, C.J. and Hill, M.J. (1984) The Policy Process in the Modern Capitalist State. Wheatsheaf Books, Brighton

Hammersley, M., and Atkinson, P. (1982) Ethnography: Principles in Practice, Tavistock, London

Harrison, S. (1981) 'The Politics of Health Manpower', in Long, A.F. and Mercer, G.(eds.), Manpower Planning in the National Health Service, Gower Press, Farnborough

Harrison, S., Pohlman, C.E., and Mercer, G. (1984) Concepts of Clinical Freedom Amongst English Physicians, Paper presented at European Association of Programmes in Health Services Studies Conference on Clinical Freedom, King's Fund, 5 June

Harrison, S. and Rathwell, T. (1980) 'The Use of Staffing Norms - a Cautionary View', Health Services Manpower Review, vol. 6. no. 4, November, pp. 9-10

Harrison, S. (1984) 'General Managers for the NHS: Substance or Symbol?', Radical Community Medicine, Spring, pp. 29-30

Hart, J.T. (1983) 'To Whom Are We Answerable?', The Lancet, November 12, pp. 1132-1133

Haywood, S.C., and Alaszewski, A. (1980) Crisis in the National Health Service: The Politics of Management, Croom Helm, London

Haywood, S.C. (1983) District Health Authorities in Action, University of Birmingham Health Services Management Centre, Research Report no. 19, Birmingham

Henderson, J.M. and Quandt, R.E. (1971) Micro-Economic Theory: A Mathmetical Approach, McGraw-Hill and Kogakusha, Tokyo, 2nd edition

Hill, M.J. (1981) 'Front-Line Administrators: Policy Implementers or the Real Policy Makers?', paper given at the Royal Institute of Public Administration Conference, April 10-11

Hiller, M.D. (ed.) (1981) Medical Ethics and the Law, Implications for Public Policy, Ballinger Publishing Company, Cambridge MA

Holland, W.W. (1983) 'Concepts and Meaning in Evaluation of Health Care', in Holland, W.W. (ed.) 1983, The Evaluation of Health Care, Oxford University Press, Oxford

Horngren, C.T. (1977) Cost Accounting: A Managerial Emphasis, PHI, New Jersey, 4th edition

Hunt, S.M. and McEwen, J. (1980) 'The Development of a Subjective Health Indicator', Sociology of Health and Illness, vol. 2, pp. 231-46

Hunt, S.M., McEwen, J., and McKenna, S.P. (1984) 'Perceived Health: Age and Sex Comparisons in a Community', Journal of Epidemiology and Community Health, vol. 38, p. 156-60

Hunter, D.J. (1984a) 'Managing Health Care', Social Policy and Administration, vol. 18, no. 1, Spring, p. 63

Hunter, D.J. (1984b) 'NHS Management: Is Griffiths the Last Quick Fix?', Public Administration vol. 62, Spring, pp. 91-94

Hyde, A. (1984) 'Oxford's Rough Ride', Health and Social Services Journal, vol. xciv. no. 4905, July 12, p. 816

Hyman, H.H. (1982) Health Planning: A Systematic Approach, 2nd Edition, Aspen Systems, Rockville, Md

Iglehart, J.K. (1984) 'Opinion Polls on Health Care', New England Journal of Medicine, 310: 4, pp. 1616-1620, June 14

Illich, I. (1975) Medical Nemisis: The Expropriation of Health, Random House, New York

Illich, I. (1976) Limits to Medicine: Medical Nemesis - The Expropriation of Health, Marion Boyars, London

Illsley, R. (1980) Professionalism or Public Health?', The Rock Carling Fellowship, Nuffield Provincial Hospitals Trust, London

Ingram, R. (ed) (1980) Accounting in the Public Sector, Brighton Press, Salt Lake City

Jarvis, M. et al. (1984) 'Quality Assurance in Long Term Care: Sherbrooke Community Centre Model', Health Management Forum, Autumn, pp. 14-25

Johnson, T.J. (1972) Professions and Power, Macmillan, London

Joskow, P.L. (1981) Controlling Hospital Costs: The Role of Government Regulation, Massachusetts of Technology Press, Cambridge, Ma

Kahn, A.J. (1977) 'Definitions of the Task: Facts, Projections, and Inventories' in N. Gilbert and H. Specht (eds.), Planning for Social Welfare: Issues, Models and Tasks, Prentice-Hall, Englewood Cliffs

Kahn, R.L., Wolfe, D.M., Quinn, R.P., Snoek, J.D., and Rosenthal, R.A. (1964) Organisational Stress: Studies in Role Conflict and Ambiguity, John Wiley, New York

Kaprio, L. (1983) 'The Role of Health Services in Society - A European View' in J. Hallas (ed.) Challenges and Changes, Nuffield Centre for Health Services Studies, Leeds

Katz, D. and Kahn, R.L. (1978) The Social Psychology of Organisations, John Wiley, New York

Kimberly, J.R., Norling, F., and Weiss, J.A. (1983) 'Pondering the Performance Puzzle' in Hall and Quinn Organisational Theory (q.v.)

Klarman, H.E., Francis, J.O.S. and Rosenthal, G.D. (1973) 'Efficient Treatment of Patients with Kidney Failure', in Cooper, M.H. and Culyer, A.J. Health Economics, Penguin Books, Harmondsworth

Klein, R. (1977) 'Priorities and the Problems of Planning', British Medical Journal, vol. II, no. 6094, pp. 1096-1097

Klein, R.E. (1980) Ideology, Class and the National Health Service, King's Fund, Project Paper no. RC4, London

Klein, R. (1982) 'Performance, Evaluation and the NHS: A Case Study in Conceptual Perplexity and Organisational Complexity', Public Administration, vol. 60, pp. 385-407

Klein, R.E. (1983) The Politics of the National Health Service, Longman, London

Klein, R. (1984) 'Rationing Health Care', British Medical Journal, 21 July, pp. 143-4

Kleinbaum, D.G., Kupper, L.L., and Morgenstern, H., (1982) Epidemiologic Research: Principles and Quantitative Methods, Lifetime Learning Publications, Belmont, California

Korcok, M. (1983) 'The Ontario Hospital Experience: American Managers March In', Canadian Medical Association Journal, 128, March 15, pp. 698-707

Korner, E. Steering Group on Health Services Information (1982) First Report to the Secretary of State, HMSO, London

Korner, E. and Mason, A. (1983) 'A National Approach to Health Services Management Information Services', Effective Health Care, vol. I, no. 1, pp. 59-64

Lalonde, M. (1974) A New Perspective on the Health of Canadians, Government of Canada, Ottawa*

Larkin, G. (1983) Occupational Monopoly and Modern Medicine, Tavistock, London

LeClair, M. (1975) 'The Canadian Health Care System' in S. Andreopoulos (ed.) pp. 11-93

Lee, K. (1977) 'Public Expenditure, Planning and Local Democracy' in K. Barnard and K. Lee (eds), Conflicts in the National Health Service, Croom Helm, London

Bibliography

Lee, K. and Mills, A. (1979) 'The Contribution of Economics to Health Service Planning', Health and Social Services Journal, Centre Eight Papers, March

Lee, K. and Mills, A. (1982) Policy-Making and Planning in the Health Sector, Croom Helm, London

Leibenstein, H. (1966) 'Allocative Efficiency vs X-Efficiency', American Economic Review, 56, pp. 392-145, June

Lewin and Associates (1976) Government Controls on the Health Care System: The Canadian Experience, Washington DC

Lewis, A.F., and Modle, W.J. (1982) 'Health Indicators: What Are They? An Approach to Efficacy in Health Care', Health Trends, vol. 14, no. 1, pp. 3-8

Lindblom, C.E. (1959) 'The Science of Muddling Through', Public Administration Review, vol. 19, no. 3

Lindblom, C.E. (1979) 'Still Muddling, Not Yet Through' Public Administration Review, vol. 39, no. 6

Lindblom, C.E., and Cohen, D.K. (1979) Usable Knowledge: Social Science and Social Problem Solving, Yale University Press, New Haven

Lipsey, R.G. (1966) An Introduction to Positive Economics, Weidenfeld and Nicolson, London

Council for Science and Society (1982) Expensive Medical Techniques, London

London Health Planning Consortium (1979) Acute Hospital Services in London, DHSS, HMSO, London

Long, A.F. (1984) Research Into Health and Illness: Issues in Design Analysis and Practice, Gower Publishing Company, Aldershot

Love, R., Coburn, D. and Kauvert, J.A. (1984) 'Beyond Individual Accountability: Public Policy Perspectives', in D.P. Lumsden (ed.) Community Mental Health Action, Canadian Public Health Association, Ottawa, pp. 302-11

Luke, R.D., and Boss, R.W. (1981) 'Barriers Limiting the Implementation of Quality Assurance Program', Health Services Research, vol. 16, no.3, pp. 306-316

Lukes, S. (1974) Power: A Radical View, Macmillan, London

Macrae, N. (1984) 'Health Care International: Better Care at One-Eighth the Cost?', The Economist, April 28, pp. 17-33

Bibliography

Magee, C.G. and Osmolski, R. (1979) Manual of
    Procedures for Specialty Costing, Research
    Paper, University College, Cardiff
Majone, G., and Wildavsky, A. (1979) 'Implementation
    as Evolution' in Pressman and Wildavsky,
    Implementation
Manitoba, Department of Health and Social
    Development (1972) White Paper on Health
    Policy, Manitoba
Manning, W.G., Leibowitz, A., Goldberg, C.A., et al
    (1984) 'A Controlled Trial of Effect of a
    Pre-paid Group Practice on Use of Services, New
    England Journal of Medicine, 310, pp. 1505-
    1510
March, J.G. and Simon, H.A. (1959) Organisations,
    John Wiley, New York
Mather, H.G., Morgan, D.C., Pearson, N.G., Read,
    K.L.Q., Shaw, D.B., Steed, G.R., Thorne, M.G.,
    Lawrence, C.J., and Riley, I.S. (1976)
    'Myocardial Infarction: A Comparison Between
    Home and Hospital Care for Patients', British
    Medical Journal, April 17, pp. 925-9
Maxwell, R., Hardie, R., Rendall, M., Day, M.,
    Lawrence, H. and Walton, N. (1983) 'Seeking
    Quality', Lancet, January, pp. 45-48
Maxwell, R.J. (1983) 'Money and Management: The NHS
    in the 1980s', Hospital and Health Services
    Review, March, pp. 53-56
McCall, G.J., and Simons, J.L. (eds.) (1969) Issues
    in Participant Observation: A Text and Reader,
    Addison-Wesley, Reading, MA
McCarthy, M. (1982a) 'A Five Year Plan for Better
    Health', The Health Services, July 11, pp.
    14-15
McCarthy, M. (1982b) Epidemiology and Policies for
    Health Care Planning, King's Fund, Oxford
    University Press, Oxford
McCarthy, M. (1983) 'Are Efficiency Measures
    Effective?', Health and Social Services
    Journal, 15 December, pp. 1500-1501
McDermott, W. (1969) 'Demography, Culture, and
    Evoluationary Stages of Medicine' in
    E. Kibourne and W.G. Smillie (eds.) Human
    Ecology and Public Health, Macmillan,
    Toronto
McKeown, T. (1976) The Role of Medicine: Dream,
    Mirage or Nemesis?, Nuffield Provincial
    Hospitals Trust, Oxford University Press,
    Oxford

Bibliography

McNaught, A. (1981) 'The Neglect of Planning in Health Districts', <u>Hospital and Health Services Review</u>, September, pp. 241-243

Mechanic, D., (1962) 'The Concept of Illness Behaviour', <u>Journal of Disesase</u>, vol. 15, pp. 189-94

Michels, R. (1915) <u>Political Parties</u>, Constable, London

Miesel, A., (1981) 'Informed Consent: Who Decides for Whom?' in Hiller, M.D. (ed.) (1981), <u>Medical Ethics and the Law</u>, Ballinger Publishing Company, Cambridge, MA

Miettinen, O.S. (1981) <u>Epidemiology at the Discipline of Medical Occurrence Research</u>, (unpublished), Institute of Occupational Health, Helsinki, Finland

Miettinen, O.S. (1983) 'The Need for Randomisation in the Study of Intended Effects', <u>Statistics in Medicine</u>, vol. 2, pp. 267-71

Ministry of Health (1956) <u>Report of the Committee of Enquiry into the Cost of the National Health Service</u>, The Guillebaud Report, Cmnd 9663, HMSO, London

Ministry of Health (1962) <u>A Hospital Plan for England and Wales</u>, HMSO, London

Mooney, G.H. (1983) <u>Marginal Analysis, or Asking the Right Questions as a Way of Geting to the Right Answers</u>, Paper presented to Chairman's Conference, National Association of Health Authorities, 3-4 March

Mooney, G.H., Russell, E.M. and Weir, R.D. (1980) <u>Choices for Health Care</u>, Macmillan, London

Morris, J.N. (1982) 'Epidemiology and Prevention', <u>Millbank Memorial Fund Quarterly/Health and Society</u>, vol. 60, no. 1, pp. 1-16

Mosca, G. (1939) <u>The Ruling Class</u>, McGraw-Hill, London

Mowbray, D. (1983a) 'Management Advisory Service: The Oxford and South Western Region-Wide Experiment', <u>Hospital and Health Services Review</u>, September, pp. 207-21

Mowbray, D. (1983b) 'Just What are we Trying to Achieve?' <u>Health and Social Services Journal</u>, 15 September, pp. 1110-1111

Muir Gray, J.A. (1977) 'The Failure of Preventive Medicine', <u>The Lancet</u>, 24 & 31 December, pp. 1338-9

NHS Management Inquiry (1983) Letter to Secretary of State, 6 October, ('<u>The Griffiths Report</u>')

Navarro, V. (1976) 'Social Class, Political Power and the State and Their Implications in Medicine', Social Science and Medicine, vol. 8, no. 2, pp. 179-216

Neuhauser, D. (1983) 'DRGs in Jersey', Effective Health Care, vol. 1, no. 3

Newhouse, J.P. et al (1982) Some Interim Results from a Controlled Trial of Cost Sharing in Health Insurance, RAND Corporation, Santa Monica

Niebuhr, R. (1945) The Children of Light and the Children of Darkness, Misbetelo, London

Office of Population Censuses and Surveys (OPCS) (1983) General Household Survey 1981, HMSO London

Oldham, P.D., and Newell, D.J. (1977) 'Fluoridation of Water Supplies and Cancer - A Possible Association', Applied Statistics, vol. 2, pp. 125-35

Oliver, M.F. (1983) 'Should We Not Forget About Mass Control of Coronary Risk Factors?', The Lancet, 2 July, pp. 37-8

Olson, M. (1965) The Logic of Collective Action: Public Goods and the Theory of Groups, Harvard University Press, Cambridge

Ontario, Government (1970) Report of the Committee on the Healing Arts, Queen's Printer, Toronto

Ontario, Ministry of Health (1983) 'Health Care: The 80s and Beyond', Ministry of Health Toronto

Ontario, Ministry of Health (1984a) Interim Policy and Guidelines for Geriatric Day Hospitals in Ontario, Ministry of Health, Toronto

Ontario, Ministry of Health (1984b) Guidelines and Submission Procedures for the Community Health Care Program, Ministry of Health, Toronto

Oxford RHA, 'The Region's Health - A New Way Forward (published in June 1984)

Oxford RHA (1982) 'Implications for the Oxford Region of Current Government Policy: A Paper for Information, Discussion and Consultation in the Oxford Region'

Oxford RHA (1984) press release, 'Taking a Spirited Look at the Future', quoted in Hospital and Health Services News and Appointments Review, no. 170, 8-15 February

Palmer, S., West, P., Patrick, D. and Glynn, M. (1979) 'Mortality Indices in Resource Allocation', Community Medicine, vol. I, pp. 275-281

Pannenborg, C.O., Van der Werff, A., Hirsch, G., and Barnard, K.A. (eds) (1984) Re-orienting Health Services: Application of a Systems Approach, Plenum Press, New York

Pareto, W. (1972) Manual of Political Economy, Translated by A.S. Schivier and A.N. Page, Macmillan, London

Pauly, M.V. (1972) Medical Care at Public Expense, Praeger, New York

Perrin, J.R. (1978) Capital Maintenance and Allocation in the Health Service, University of Warwick, Occasional Paper, April

Peters, B.G., Doughtie, J.C., and McCullough, K.M. (1978) 'Do Public Policies Vary in Different Types of Democratic System?' in Lewis, P.G., Potter, D.C., and Castles, F.G. The Practice of Comparative Politics, Longman and Open University Press, London

Peters, T.J. and Waterman, R.H. (1982) In Search of Excellence, Harper and Row, New York

Pfeffer, J. and Salancik, G.R. (1978) The External Control of Organisations: A Resource Dependence Perspective, Harper and Row, New York

Pfeffer, J. (1981) Power in Organisations, Pitman, Marshfield

Pfeffer, J. (1982) Organisations and Organisation Theory, Pitman, Boston

Piachaud, D. and Weddell, J.M. (1972) 'The Economics of Treating Varicose Veins', International Journal of Epidemiology, vol. 1, no. 1, pp. 287-294

Poggi, G. (1965) 'A Main Theme of Contemporary Sociological Analysis: Its Achievements and Limitations', British Journal of Sociology, vol. 16

Polanyi, M. (1966) The Tacit Dimension, Doubleday and Co. Ltd., New York

Popper, K.R. (1972) Objective Knowledge, Oxford University Press, Oxford

Pressman, J.L., and Wildavsky, A. (1979) Implementation: How Great Expectations in Washington are Dashed in Oakland, University of California Press, Berkeley

Prest, A.R. and Turvey, R. (1965) 'Cost Benefit Analysis: A Review', Economic Journal, December

Pugh, D.S., and Hickson, D.J. (1976) Organisation Structure in its Context, Saxon House, Farnborough

Quebec, Government (1966-70) Report of the Commission of Inquiry on Health and Social Welfare, 7 vol.s (Castonguay-Nepveu Report) Official publisher, Government of Quebec

Rathwell, T.A. (1981) 'Politics of Persuasion', Times Health Supplement, 18 December

Rathwell, T.A. (1984) 'Health Services Planning - Observation of the Relationship Between Theory and Practice' in M. Clarke (ed.) London Papers 13: Planning and Analysis in Health Care Systems, Pion, London

Rathwell, T.A. and Barnard, K. (1983) NHS Management Enquiry - A New Management Era, Report of A One-Day Conference, Nuffield Centre for Health Services Studies, University of Leeds

Renaud, M. (1975) 'On the Structural Constraints to State Intervention in Health', International Journal of Health Services, 5, 4, pp. 559-71

Renaud, M. (1981) 'Reform or Illusion? An Analysis of the Quebec State Intervention in Health', in D. Coburn et al (eds) Canadian Health Services, pp. 369-92

Richardson, J.J., and Jordan, A.G. (1979) Governing Under Pressure: The Policy Process in a Post-Parliamentary Democracy, Martin Robertson, Oxford

Richardson, T. (1984) 'Under the Banyan Tree', The Lancet, 31 March

Rivlin, A.M. (1977) 'The Planning, Programming and Budgetting System in the Department of Health, Education and Welfare: Some Lessons from Experience' in Planning for Social Welfare (ed.) N. Gilbert and H. Specht, Prentice-Hall, Englewood Cliffs, NJ

Roberts, F. (1952) The Cost of Health, Turnstile Press, London

Roberts, G. (1983) quoted in Hospital and Health Services News and Appointments Review, no. 142, 5-12 January

Robinson, J. (1933) The Economics of Imperfect Competition, MacMillan, London

Rodwin, V.G. (1984) The Heath Planning Predicament, University of California Press, Berkeley, USA

Roemer, M.I. (1976) Health Care Systems in World Perspective, Health Administration Press, Ann Arbor

Rohrbaugh, J. (1983) 'The Competing Values Approach' in Hall and Quinn Organisational Theory (q.v.)

Romeder, J.M, and McWhinnie, J.R. (1977) 'Potential Years of Life Lost Between Ages 1 to 70: An Indicator of Premature Mortality for Health Planning', International Journal of Epidemiology, vol. 6, no 2, pp. 143-51

Roos, N.P., Gaumont, M. and Horne, J.M. (1976) 'The Impact of Physician Surplus on the Distribution of Physicians across Canada', Canadian Public Policy, 2, pp. 169-91

Rose, M. (1978) Industrial Behaviour, Penguin Books, Harmondsworth

Rose, R. (1976) Managing Presidential Objectives, Free Press, New York

Rosser, R. (1982) 'Health Indicators: Psychometric Studies of the Severity of Illness', in CASPE Research, Output Measurement for Health Services, King's Fund Centre, London, pp. 35-45

Rosser, R.M., and Watts, V.C. (1972) 'The Measurement of Hospital Output', International Journal of Epidemiology, vol. 1, pp. 361-8

Rosser, R.M., and Watts, V.C. (1978) 'The Measurement of Illness', Journal of Operational Research Society, vol. 29, no. 6, pp. 529-40

Royal Commission on the National Health Service (1979) Report, Cmnd 7615, HMSO, London

Rutstein, D.D. (1974) Blueprints for Medical Care, MIT Press, Cambridge

Rutstein, D.D., Berenberg, W., Chalmers, T.C., Child, C.G., Fishman, A.P., and Perrin, E.B. (1976) 'Measuring the Quality of Medical Care: A Clinical Method', New England Journal of Medicine, 11 March, pp. 582-8

Rutstein, D.D. et al (1980) 'Measuring the Quality of Medical Care: Second Revision of Tables of Indexes', (correspondence), New England Journal of Medicine, 15 May, p. 1146

Ryant, J.C. (1977) 'The Integration of Services in Rural and Urban Communities' Canadian Journal of Social Work Education, 2, 3

Salaman, G. (1979) Work Organisations: Resistance and Control, Longman, London

Saltman, R.B., and Young, D.W. (1981) 'The Hospital Power Equilibrium: An Alternative View of the Cost Containment Dilemma', Journal of Health Politics, Policy and Law, vol. 6, no. 3, Fall

Sapsford, R.J., and Evans, J. (1979) Evaluation of Research, DE304 Research Methods in Education and the Social Sciences, Block 8, Open University Press, Milton Keynes

Scheckler, W., and Schulz, R. (forthcoming) The
Transformation of Health Services in Dane
County, University of Wisconsin, Madison

Schon, D.A. (1971) Beyond the Stable State, Temple
Smith, London

Schulz, R.I., Greenley, J.R., and Peterson, R.W.
(1983) 'Management Cost, and Quality of Acute
Inpatient Psychiatric Services', Medical Care,
vol. 21, no. 9, September

Schulz, R.I., and Harrison, S. (1983) Teams and Top
Managers in the National Health Services: A
Survey and a Strategy, King's Fund Project
Paper no. 41, London

Schulz, R.I., and Johnson, A.C. (1983) The
Management of Hospitals, McGraw-Hill, New
York

Schumacher, F. (1974) Small is Beautiful: Towards a
Theory of Large Scale Organisation, Sphere
Books, London

Scott, W.R., Flood, A., and Ewy, W. (1979)
'Organisational Determinants of Services,
Quality, and Cost of Care in Hospitals',
Milbank Memorial Fund Quarterly, 57: 234

Scrivens, E. and Charlton, J. (1983) 'Warning
Lights?', Health and Social Services Journal,
15 December, pp. 1501-1502

Senn, S.J. and Shaw, H. (1978) 'Some Problems in
Applying the National Formula to Area and
District Revenue Allocations', Journal of
Epidemiology and Community Health, vol. 32,
pp. 22-27

Shepherd, W. (1979) The Economics of Industrial
Organisation, PHI, New Jersey

Shortell, S.M., Becker, S., and Neuhauser, D. (1976)
'The Effects of Management Practices on
Hospital Efficiency and Quality of Care', in
Shortell, S.M., and Brown, M. (eds)
Organisation Research in Hospitals, Blue Cross
Association, Chicago

Silverman, D. (1970) The Theory of Organisations,
Heinemann Educational Books, London

Simon, H.A. (1957) Administrative Behaviour,
Macmillan, New York

Simon, H.A. (1959) 'Theories of Decision Making in
Economics and Behavioural Science', American
Economic Review, XLIV, June

Slayton, P. and Trebilock, M.J. (1978) (eds) The
Professions and Public Policy, University of
Toronto Press, Toronto

Bibliography

Smith, P., and Haggard, S. (1982) 'Planning for a Single Specialty in a Health District', Journal of the Operational Research Society, vol. 33, p. 29-39

Soderstrom, L. (1978) The Canadian Health Care System, Croom Helm, London

Sox, H.C. (1979) 'Quality of Patient Care by Nurse Practitioners and Physicians' Assistants: A Ten Year Perspective', Annals of Internal Medicine, 91, 459-68

Stacey, M. (1977) 'A Survey of Concepts of Health and Disease', in SSRC Health and Social Policy, Appendix III, HMSO, London

Stallones, R.A. (1983) 'Mortality and the Multiple Risk Factor Intervention Trial', American Journal of Epidemiology, vol. 117, no. 6, pp. 647-50

Starr, P. (1982) The Social Transformation of American Medicine, Basic Books, New York

Steele, R.A. and Dingwall-Fordyce, I. (1983) 'Equity and an Equal Opportunity for Treatment' Hospital and Health Services Review, May, pp. 126-128

Steering Group on Health Service Information (1982) Report, HMSO, London

Stern, P.C. (1979) Evaluating Social Science Research, Oxford University Press, New York

Stevenson, G. (1977) 'Federalism and the Political Economy of the Canadian State', in L. Panitch (ed.) The Canadian State, University of Toronto Press, Toronto, pp. 71-100

Stewart, G.T. (1984) 'Some Thoughts on Griffiths', Lancet, 24 March, pp. 672-2

Stonich, P. (ed.) (1982) Implementing Strategy: Making Strategy Happen, Ballinger, Cambridge

Susser, M. (1974) 'Ethical Components in the Definition of Health', International Journal of Health Services, vol. 4, no. 3, pp. 539-48

Tatchell, M. (1983) 'Measuring Hospital Output: A Review of the Service Mix and Case Mix Approaches', Social Science and Medicine, vol. 17, no. 13, pp. 871-833

Taylor, M.G. (1960) 'The Role of the Medical Profession in the Formulation and Execution of Public Policy', Canadian Journal of Economics and Political Science, 26, 1, pp. 108-27

Taylor, M.G. (1978) Health Insurance and Canadian Public Policy, McGill-Queen's University Press, Montreal

The Health Services (1983) 'Joint Care for the
    Elderly: A THS Special Supplement', The Health
    Services, 23 September
Thompson, F.J. (1981) Health Policy and the
    Bureaucracy, Massachusetts Institute of
    Technology Press, London
Thompson, J.D. and Tuden, A. (1959) 'Strategies,
    Structures and Processes of Organisational
    Decision' in J.D. Thompson et al (eds)
    Comparative Studies in Administration,
    University of Pittsburgh Press, Pittsburgh, Pa
Tisdell, C.A. (1982) Micro-Economics of Markets,
    John Wiley, Brisbane
Tomkins, C. (1983) The Effect of Political and
    Economic Changes (1974-82) on Financial
    Control Processes in Some UK Local Authorities,
    University of Bath Research Paper
Torrance, G.M. (1981) 'Socio-historical Overview',
    in D. Coburn et al (eds) Health and Canadian
    Society, pp. 13-19
Townsend, P., and Davidson, N. (1982) Inequalities
    in Health, Penguin Books, Harmondsworth
Tsai, S.P., Lee, E.S., and Hardy, R.J. (1978) 'The
    Effect of a Reduction in Leading Causes of
    Death: Potential Gains in Life Expectancy',
    American Journal of Public Health, vol. 68, no.
    10, pp. 966-71
Tsai, S.P., Lee, E.S., and Kautz, J.A. (1982)
    'Changes in Life Expenctancy in the United
    States Due to Decline in Mortality, 1969-
    1975', American Journal of Epidemiology, vol.
    116, no. 2, pp. 376-84
Tsalikis, G. (1982a) 'The Consequences of Canadian
    Health Care Policy', in Canadian Council on
    Social Development 'Issues in Canadian Social
    Policy, vol. II
Tsalikis, G. (1982b) 'Canada', in Hokenstad, M.C.
    and Ritvo, R.A. (eds) Linking Health Care and
    Social Services, Sage Publications, Beverly
    Hills, USA, pp. 125-61
Tuohy, C. (1976) 'Medical Politics after Medicare:
    The Ontario Case', Canadian Public Policy, 2,
    Spring, pp. 192-210
University of British Columbia Health Policy Study
    Group (1982) 'Current Issues in Health Policy
    Making for the Government of British Columbia',
    Health Management Forum, 3,3, pp. 27-86

Van T'Hoff, W. (1981) 'Report of Results of an Inquiry Conducted by Questions About Audit', Paper given at a Conference of the Royal College of Physicians of London, 23 January: reported in The Lancet, 30 January

Vayda, E. (1983) 'Aspects of Medical Manpower under National Health Insurance in Canada', Journal of Public Health Policy, December, pp. 504-13

Vayda, E. and Deber R.B. (1984) 'The Canadian Health Care System: An Overview', Social Science and Medicine, 18, 3, pp. 191-97

Vickers, G. (1965) The Art of Judgement, Chapman and Hall, London

Vuori, H.Y. (1982) Quality Assurance of Health Services: Concepts and Methodologies, Public Health in Europe 16, Regional Office for Europe, World Health Organisation, Copenhagen

Wadsworth, M.E.J. (1971) Health And Sickness: The Choice of Treatment, Tavistock Press, London

Walters, B. (1982) 'State, Capital and Labour: The Introduction of Federal-Provincial Insurance for Physician Care in Canada', Canadian Review of Sociology and Anthropology, 19, 2, pp. 157-72

Weber, M. (1947) The Theory of Social and Economic Organisation, trans. Henderson, A.M. and Parsons, T., Free Press, New York

Weed, L.L. (1973) 'Quality Control', in Hurst, J.W. and Walker, H.J. (eds) (1973) Applying the Problem - Oriented System, Medcom Press, New York

Weisbrod, B. (1982) 'A Guide to Benefit-Cost Analysis, as seen through a Controlled Equipment in Treating the Mentally Ill', Journal of Health Politics, Policy and Law, vol. 7, no. 4

Weller, G.R. (1980) 'The Determinants of Canadian Health Policy', Journal of Health Politics, Policy and Law, 5, 3, pp. 405-18

Weller, G.R. and Manga, P. (1983) 'The Development of Health Policy in Canada', in M.M. Atkinson and M.A. Chandler (eds) The Politics of Canadian Public Policy, University of Toronto Press, Toronto, pp. 223-46

Wickings, I. (1983) 'Consultants Face the Figures', Health and Social Services Journal, 8 December

Williams, A. (1974) 'Measuring the Effectiveness of Health Care Systems', British Journal of Preventive and Social Medicine, vol. 28, pp. 196-202

Bibliograpy

Williams, J.N. and Brook R.H. (1978) 'Quality
    Measurement and Assurance', Health and Medical
    Care Services, 1: 3, pp. 1-15, May/June
Winslow, G.R. (1982) Triage and Justice, University
    of Californai Press, London
Winyard, G.P.A. (1981) 'RAWP - New Injustice for
    Old', British Medical Journal, vol. 283, pp.
    930-932
World Health Organisation (1981) Managerial Process
    for National Health Development: Guiding
    Principles, Geneva
Yates, J. (1982) Hospital Beds: A Problem for
    Diagnosis and Management, Heinneman Medical,
    London
Yates, J. (1983) 'When will the Players get
    Involved?' Health and Social Services Review,
    15 September, pp. 1111-1112

objectives
    of health services
    29, 52, 126, 195,
    202, 210, 227, 236
    outcome 15, 40-1 67,
    203, 213, 233
    and Donabedian 6-7,
    227
    and need 15, 16, 52
    data on 39, 44
    evaluation 38, 46,
    142
    measures of 23, 26,
    32
    mortality as
    measures of 23-4,
    26, 28, 201
    process outcome 17
    product outcome 17
    target 16
    see also health,
    health status
Oxford Region 87-104
    passim

paradoxical effects 39,
    229
pathogenic model 21,
    24, 32
peer review 85, 86,
    192, 203, 213, 219
performance 2, 5, 79,
    122, 189, 196
    concepts of 123
    indicators 4, 142-7
    see also performance
    review
performance review 1,
    47, 142
    aims 5, 7
    environment of 4
    see also
    performance
planning for health
    care 130-38, 170,
    173, 189, 192-5,
    207, 226, 228
pluralistic model 112-
    5, 121, 123, 218-9
    see also
    implementation

power 112-3, 118, 123,
    153, 165, 218-9, 225
practitioners 5, 7, 15,
    23, 28, 31, 44, 47, 48,
    165, 180, 182
private practice 84-5, 90,
    164-6, 182, 189
process 17, 46, 67, 213
    and Donabedian 6-7,
    189, 202, 227
    see also outcome,
    structure
producer sovereignty 58,
    63, 153, 194, 232
professional autonomy 197,
    199, 214, 219, 229, 235

quality assurance 2, 47,
    199,
    and quality assessment
    2, 203, 214
    barriers to 3
    environment of 4
quality of care 23, 26,
    38, 207
    definition 3, 5, 15,
    214
    interpersonal aspect 4,
    7, 14
    principle of 3
    technical aspect 4, 14
    types of 6

randomisation 42, 50
randomised controlled
    trial 42, 46, 50
rational decision making
    44, 72, 104, 159, 179,
    185, 194, 105, 237
rationality 107, 108, 112,
    113
rationing 77, 91, 93, 218,
    231, 238
resource allocation 62,
    134-8, 186-8, 227-8
reliability 24, 29, 37,
    38, 44, 49, 52
reorganisation of NHS 61,
    87, 129-30, 239-40

sensitivity 37, 38, 42,

LIST OF CONTRIBUTORS

Andrew F Long
Lecturer in Quantitative Methods
The Nuffield Centre
Department of Social Policy and
   Health Services Studies
University of Leeds
England

Stephen Harrison
Lecturer in Health Services Organisation
The Nuffield Centre

Jack Hallas
Lecturer in Policy Studies
The Nuffield Centre

Tom Rathwell
Lecturer in Health Planning
The Nuffield Centre

Keith Barnard
Senior Lecturer in Health Planning
The Nuffield Centre

Geoffrey Mercer
Lecturer in Sociology
Department of Sociology
University of Leeds
England

Ray Brooks
Director of Financial Management Programmes
The Management Centre
University of Bradford
England

List of Contributors

Rockwell Schulz
Professor of Preventive Medicine
Director of Programs in Health
  Services Administration
University of Wisconsin
Madison
USA